STUTTERING

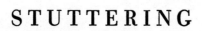

STUTTERING

A New Look at an Old Problem
Based on Neurophysiological Aspects

By

CHARLES P. OVERSTAKE, Ph.D.

*Director
Wichita Speech Science Laboratory
Formerly, Chairman and Head Speech Pathologist
Neurological Diagnostic Unit
Director of Professional Services
Institute of Logopedics
Wichita, Kansas
Assistant Professor in Logopedics
Wichita State University
Wichita, Kansas*

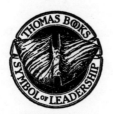

CHARLES C THOMAS • **PUBLISHER**
Springfield • *Illinois* • *U.S.A.*

Published and Distributed Throughout the World by
CHARLES C THOMAS • PUBLISHER
BANNERSTONE HOUSE
301-327 East Lawrence Avenue, Springfield, Illinois, U.S.A.

© *1979, by* CHARLES C THOMAS • PUBLISHER
ISBN 0-398-03896-1
Library of Congress Catalog Card Number: 78 20664

With THOMAS BOOKS *careful attention is given to all details of manufacturing and design. It is the Publisher's desire to present books that are satisfactory as to their physical qualities and artistic possibilities and appropriate for their particular use.* THOMAS BOOKS *will be true to those laws of quality that assure a good name and good will.*

616.8554
O96
—

Printed in the United States of America
N-11

Library of Congress Cataloging in Publication Data

Overstake, Charles P.
    Stuttering : a new look at an old problem based on neurophysiological aspects.

    Bibliography: p.
    Includes index.
    1. Stuttering. 2. Neurophysiology. I. Title. [DNLM: 1. Stuttering. 2. Neurophysiology. WM475.3096s]
    RC424.093   616.8'554'071   78-20664
    ISBN 0-398-03896-1

PREFACE

THE ENTIRE WORLD is aware of stuttering; it occurs in almost every language. The existence of this problem has been recognized for centuries. Scientists, researchers, philosophers, physicians, and the man on the street have wondered about the enigma and why it occurs. In spite of all the interest and effort expended toward a better understanding, it still remains a mystery.

The author was curious about and intrigued with the problem of stuttering long before he became a speech pathologist. The questions were ever present. Why do people stutter? Are they ill? Is this an indication of an emotional problem, or brain damage, or what?

In spite of information garnered from many college courses in stuttering and speech science, the problem still remained unexplained to this author's satisfaction. There were many theories and hypotheses being circulated. Every conceivable cause seemed to have been proffered, and yet no one seemed to be willing to say that a particular theory was the correct one. The authorities differed in their explanations of the underlying ramifications.

Because of the apparent uncertainty of most individuals in the field of speech and hearing, this author began his own investigation of the problem. All theories and conjectures were read and deciphered. They all tended to focus on one aspect or another of difficulty, but not on the total problem with its varying symptoms. The author followed other leads. For example, a close friend with cerebral palsy, athetoid in type, stuttered profusely. Were stutterers persons who had mild athetosis with only the speech affected? That idea did not seem neurologically reasonable. The search continued over many years. The author examined hundreds of stutterers at every age level. Questions

v

were asked and behaviors observed. Many hypotheses were
formulated and then abandoned.

As the years passed and more information was garnered, it
seemed to become increasingly evident that the problem had to
be of a neurophysiological or organic origin. All avenues led in
that direction. If the problem were emotional, psychotic, or
neurotic in nature, there would have to be involvement of the
limbic nervous system, the emotional control system of human
beings. Did the problem involve the endocrine system because
of its relationship to the hypothalamus and the limbic system?
These concepts were explored and deferred for a better answer.

All human motor behaviors are neuromuscular functions.
Speech output is neuromuscular behavior. Breathing requires
the same type of muscular activity. Laryngeal functions and the
articulation for speech are all muscle patterns designed to produce different sounds. They have to function in patterned form.
A person does not have to think about muscle patterns when he
talks. It just happens. A thought occurs and speech results.
How, how does it come about?

Courses taken in neurology, and neurophysiology, and kinesiology failed to provide satisfactory answers. The author then
had the good fortune to teach neurology and neurophysiology at
university level. The old saying became very true: "If you
really want to learn a subject, teach it." It was at this time that
the function of the cerebellum became intriguing to the author.
Further study revealed some possible involvement of this part of
the cerebellum and its relationship to patterned muscle behaviors. If the cerebellum is involved with patterned muscle behaviors, it has to include the muscles used in speech. Here may lie
the answers to some speech disorders, including stuttering.

This book has been based on the strong belief that the nervous system holds the key to the problem of stuttering. The
cerebral cortex and the cerebellum are involved; they almost have
to be because of their involvement in the total motor functioning
of human beings.

After a review of the prevailing literature, the theory presented here is a new look at the old problem of stuttering. Some

authorities appear to have come very close to the correct answers. It is this author's wish that the new look may come even closer to answering questions concerning this speech disorder.

If the new look provides acceptable answers to many of the primary questions concerning stuttering, then the therapeutic programs suggested in this writing may initiate further research. Therapy programs may also be developed for the remission of stuttering in those who are so oppressed by its effects on themselves and their loved ones.

The author sincerely desires that all who read this book, regardless of their beliefs, professions, or problems, will profit from what has been presented. It is realized that the concepts introduced will be closely examined, completely dissected, and highly criticized; it must be done. May what has been written here stand the test, or at least stimulate new thinking and research to find the true cause of and to eliminate stuttering.

Grateful thanks and respect are extended to all authors who graciously permitted this author to quote and paraphrase their works. They have toiled arduously to search out and present their views. The author trusts that he has submitted their works adequately and has acknowledged them satisfactorily.

Others have helped and given enthusiastically of their time and capabilities. Appreciation is due to Mr. Clyde Berger and his staff in the library of the Institute of Logopedics for their cooperation and work in searching out information requested by the author. Also, the author is grateful to Mrs. Carol E. Ross for her critical reviews and grammatical assistance, and to Mrs. Ruth Vawter Rankin for her editing competence and assistance in finalizing this manuscript.

In closing, this book is dedicated to all the persons in the world who stutter. May it prove beneficial to all of you. And to little *"Muffin"* and all the small infants everywhere who do not stutter, may they never experience this enigma, perhaps because of what has been written here.

CONTENTS

Page

Preface v

Chapter

1. OPENING THE DISCUSSION 3
   Definition of Stuttering 7
   Comparison of Stuttering and Normal Speech 9
   Concerning the Author's Theory 10
   Summary 13
2. PREVAILING THEORIES 14
   Stuttering As a Learned Behavior 14
   Stuttering As a Result of Psychoneurotic or
       Psychological Conflict 19
   Stuttering As the Result of a Neurological or
       Physiological Variation 23
   Summary 34
3. CURRENTLY RECOGNIZED THERAPEUTIC PROCEDURES 35
   Summary 49
4. STUTTERING IS A SYNDROME 50
   Stuttering Blocks 51
   Hypertonus 53
   Emotions 54
   Secondary Symptoms 54
   Stuttering versus Cluttering 56
   Summary 58
5. A NEW LOOK AT THE OLD PROBLEM 59
   Summary 75
6. THE ESTABLISHMENT OF MORE NORMAL SPEECH BEHAVIOR . 76

Chapter   *Page*

Breathing 87

Articulation of Speech 101

Rate of Speech 102

Reading 104

Secondary Symptoms 104

Thinking Aloud 106

Extending Propositional Levels 108

Normal Fluency and Nonfluency 109

Emotions 110

Postscript 111

Summary 113

7. MAINTENANCE OF ESTABLISHED NORMAL COMMUNICATION

AND ETC. 114

Monitoring 116

Delayed Auditory Feedback 117

Childhood Nonfluency 118

Outline of Possible Therapy Sessions for Stuttering ... 123

Speech Problems Resulting from Cerebellar Damage .. 125

Future Study 126

Summary and Conclusions 129

Glossary 133

References 136

Index 139

STUTTERING

Chapter 1

OPENING THE DISCUSSION

N o speech problem has received so much attention over such an extended period of time as stuttering. This puzzling riddle appears to have defied exploration for centuries and has refused to yield its secret. It is the oldest speech problem noted in the history of speech and language. Stuttering has demoralized those who have suffered from it. It appears that ever since the onset of the problem there have been those who have searched in vain for a remedy or therapeutic procedure to eliminate the repetitions, hesitations, prolongations, and stoppages that occur while speaking. To this day no one has completely solved this enigma that plagues so many human beings.

Historically, stuttering dates back to the period before Christ. During the era before Christ, Herodotus (464–424 BC), Hippocrates (450–375 BC), and Aristotle (384–322 BC) were noted to have mentioned the problem and, in some instances suggested a remedy. In Biblical times, Moses complained to the Lord that he could not lead the Children of Israel because he was slow of speech and of a slow tongue; stuttering? (Exodus 4:10). Galen (AD 166) talked about stuttering. He blamed the tongue and suggested it be cauterized as a cure.

Stuttering apparently was known during the existence of the Kingdom of the Divine Pharaohs, Egypt (3200 BC–AD 300). It has been reported that there is reference to the problem in their ancient hieroglyphics. Since those early times, stuttering has been a problem that has brought disgrace and internal turmoil to those who have been so afflicted.

Throughout history, many men and women have not been

3

able to achieve their potentials and live peaceful lives because of stuttering problems. In this modern day, when people should be more informed and more tolerant of all types of handicaps, they continue to abhor the problem of stuttering.

In spite of the attention that has been given to the problem of stuttering, no one to date appears to have discovered the etiology for its occurrence. Authorities in speech pathology, medicine, psychology, and related fields have proffered their thinking and the results of their research. Most will agree that the onset of nonfluent speech occurs between the ages of two and four years. Although many varying possibilities have been suggested, no one seems certain why it occurs.

Suggested causes for stuttering have come from various interested professions. Psychiatrists suggest that the problem results from a neurosis or a psychotic conflict. Psychologists infer that the onset is due to an emotional conflict and an inability to respond adequately because of a neurosis. Some speech pathologists have stated that the inception is due to the child trying to speak in sentences before he is ready for such behavior. A few speech scientists have suggested that the outbreak of nonfluency is neurologically based and may be due to such causes as cerebral dominance confusion, a lack of cortical myelinization, a possible metabolic imbalance, or delayed auditory feedback. There have been a limited number of individuals who have related the cause of the problem to one or more of the symptoms of stuttering, such as a breathing problem or rapidity of speech.

While the onset of nonfluent speech occurs between the ages of two and four years, most children develop normal fluent speech by the age of five or six. This phenomenon is also not readily understood. Some authorities have advised that a change to fluent speaking behavior occurred because a child had not been labeled a stutterer, or he overcame his emotional problems. Other persons advise that some children overcame their problems because they did not develop guilt feelings about their repetitive speech. However, a small percentage of children do not discontinue their nonfluent speech and continue to stutter.

Authorities have presented numerous reasons for the continuation of nonfluent speech. Some persons have stated that the child has been called a stutterer; therefore, he will continue to stutter. Other persons have said that the child's neurosis or psychosis has not abated and that there is a subconscious fear that he will utter unacceptable words. Still other sources have contended that he has developed an anticipation of words and sounds on which he stutters. When these words or sounds appear during speech, anxiety occurs, and the child or the adult will stutter. There are those who have said that stuttering is just a bad habit or that it really does not happen. It can be readily recognized that there have been many possible causes advanced for the continuation of this speech disorder. The question arises, Who is correct? Or, are any of the authorities completely correct in their assumptions? Perhaps this manuscript will offer some thoughts and information that will lead toward a better understanding of the total picture of stuttering.

The development of acceptable and normal speaking behaviors in individuals with speech and language defects, including stuttering, has received abundant attention. Today there are overwhelming quantities of varying therapeutic procedures being offered by those in the field of speech and hearing and in other professions in the hope of eliminating problems and improving speaking behaviors. Most of the therapies advanced are based on psychological premises, or stimulus-response behavior. Much of the therapy utilized is founded on Pavlovian or classical conditioning, which emphasizes a stimulus-response-reward system. Much emphasis is being placed on behavior modification as a newer entity in controlling human behavior and bringing about desired changes.

It seems unlikely that adequate therapeutic procedures or remedies have been developed for the correction of nonfluent speech because there is a definite lack of agreement as to the cause or etiology of stuttering and its continuation beyond the years when it should have ceased to be a problem. Most therapies used are based on the philosophy held by the individual pathologist providing the program for the correction of stuttering.

The treatment programs directed toward the alleviation of

nonfluent speech are quite diversified and numerous. ⌈ One program that receives consideration is adaptation. This procedure
is based on the concept that the individual will reduce his tendency to stutter because of increased familiarization with the
words he uses, the persons to whom he speaks, and the situations
in which he finds himself. He adapts to the speaking event; thus,
his speech is more fluent.⌉ Another therapy used is an auditory
or imitation approach in which the person hears fluent speech.
He is supposed to imitate the normal fluent speech that he hears
and to use it. There are some therapists who use a reward system for good speech in conjunction with this program.

Programs for the alleviation of stuttering take on varying
modes. It is suggested by some persons that the stutterer speak
to the beat of a metronome, that this will set a rate of speaking
and make him more fluent. Others recommend finger tapping
or hand movements to achieve the same results. A few speech
clinics use videotape and sound tracks in their programs. The
person who stutters is filmed, and his speech is recorded. This
recording is played back for him to see and to hear. He notes
his behaviors, and with each refilming and recording, he is to
correct the problems noted and speak more fluently. There are
those who use tape recorders. They tape the subject's speech
and let him hear the playback. Again, he is to listen to how he
is talking and perform in certain ways in order to improve his
rate or fluent speech output. Then, there are those therapists
who state that they just tell the person to stop stuttering.

One program that proclaims the correction of stuttering
recommends that the stutterer practice the words on which he
stutters until he does not not stutter on them anymore. Some
persons suggest that the stutterer talks too rapidly and feel that,
if he would slow down, he would talk better. There are still
others who recommend that the stutterer change his breathing
patterns when he talks, and slow down when he begins to speak,
and that this procedure will correct the problem.

There is a growing emphasis on the assumption that stuttering cannot be corrected, so the person who stutters must learn to
live with his problem. It is suggested that the stutterer learn to

stutter in a different way that may be easier and make the difficulty more palatable. In this procedure, the stutterer is supposed to be able to be selective as to the way he desires to stutter.

Psychiatrists and psychologists are stressing the elimination of the neurosis and the psychotic conflict by way of psychological consultation or psychoanalysis of the stutterer if he is an adult or an adolescent. If the person who stutters is a child, it is recommended that the parent receive the treatment. It is usually the mother who is afforded the therapy because of her affiliation with the child and the problems felt to be related to the cause of the stuttering. The child also may receive some psychological or psychiatric assistance if his problem is severe enough.

Here is a situation in which many different professionals appear to be moving in different directions to solve and to treat the same problem. Because of these diversified approaches for the correction or remediation of this speech disorder, it may be assumed that no one has truly developed an acceptable corrective therapy or treatment for the rehabilitation of stuttering behaviors.

DEFINITION OF STUTTERING

Almost everyone who has written about the problem of stuttering has provided a definition based on his interpretation of the problem. *Dorland's Medical Dictionary* (1962) states that stuttering is "a variety of faltering and interruptive speech characterized by difficulty in enunciating and joining together syllables." The dictionary also has a definition for stammering: "a faulty and interrupted manner of speech due to defects of articulation." *Dorland's* defines articulation as "the enunciation of words and sentences." If stammering is a problem characterized by a faulty or interrupted manner of articulation, and articulation is the enunciation of words, and then, if stuttering is interrupted speech characterized by difficulty in enunciation, stammering and stuttering are synonymous terms. Stuttering is used as the proper terminology for the problem in most professional areas.

Andrews and Harris (1964) have stated, "Stuttering is an in-

terruption in the normal rhythm of speech of such frequency
and abnormality as to attract attention, interfere with communication, or cause distress to a stutterer or his audience. He knows
precisely what he wishes to say, but is unable to say it because
of an involuntary repetition, prolongation or cessation of sound."
This definition is practically the same as those advanced by most
authorities, with some variations. This author would concur
with the definition, with some alterations. Further embellishments would be to include the symptoms and the characteristics
of the problem and to consider a neurophysiological basis for
the behaviors observed.

From a neurophysiological reference, the repetitions, prolongations, and cessations of sound during speaking are neuromuscular patterns. Repetitions are rapid, repetitive muscle behaviors, such as the repeating of the consonant *B* for B-B-B-B-
Bomb. During this action there are "spasms in which rigidity and
relaxation alternate in rapid succession." The quotation is the
definition for *clonus* from *Dorland's Medical Dictionary* (1962).
It would seem proper to substitute the term *clonic* for the repetitious blocks noted in stuttering since *clonic* means "in the nature
of clonus" and is in keeping with the neurophysiology of human
behavior.

In continuing with the consideration of the neuromuscular
behaviors and neurophysiology of stuttering, prolongations are
noted when a particular phoneme or vowel is produced for a
period of time beyond that considered to be normal, as *M* ——
Mom. Cessations, often referred to as stoppages, are periods
during speaking when no sound or phoneme is emitted, as in
making a *P*, during which the same position is retained. Both
of these behaviors result from "a tonic continuous contraction of
muscle due to stimulation received through the nervous system."
This is *Dorland's* (1962) definition for neurogenic tonus. Again,
it would seem to be reasonable and proper to use the term *tonic,*
meaning "characterized by continuous tension," in place of prolongation or cessation of sound.

Other neurophysiological and neuromuscular signs comprising the symptom complex called stuttering include secondary

muscle behaviors, deviant breathing patterns, and variable functioning of the cerebral cortex and cerebellum as they contribute to the total speech pattern.

Rewriting the definition of stuttering and including the foregoing additions would make it read as follows: Stuttering is a speech disorder characterized by disruptive tonic and clonic muscle behaviors and comprised of a complex of neurophysiological symptoms, which alter the normal rhythmic flow of speech to the extent that it interferes with communication and attracts attention to itself.

COMPARISON OF STUTTERING AND NORMAL SPEECH

Stuttering has been defined; now it must be noted that a stuttering person neither stutters at all times nor in every situation. There are occasions when such a person will have fluent speech. The amount of difficulty experienced is determined by the propositionality or value placed on each speaking encounter. The person who stutters can usually speak fluently while talking to himself, to close intimate friends, to animals, and while reciting rote material. He also may speak fluently when he is playing a role or acting a part. Most persons who stutter can sing fluently because singing is a different behavior and has components not found in speaking.

While stutterers can have periods of fluent speech, habitually normal, fluent speakers will encounter circumstances in which they will have problems with nonfluency. As it is with the person who stutters, the value placed on a speaking situation may be such that a problem arises. A fluent speaker may become nonfluent when he has to speak with his employer, explain a self-incriminating episode, or take the witness stand in a court of law. He also may have difficulty expressing himself when confronted with the little red light on a television camera or when speaking before a large audience. Fortunately, he only has such an experience occasionally, and his speech is fluent during his normal daily routine of work and recreation.

Explanations for these variations in speaking behaviors have been noted in the literature. The majority opinion appears to be that speakers anticipate having speech difficulties in certain situations, and as a consequence, they do. Persons who stutter are more affected by situations that are similar to those in which they previously experienced difficulty than are fluent speakers. The ability to adapt to higher levels of propositional speech is more notable within the normal speaking population.

CONCERNING THE AUTHOR'S THEORY

As noted earlier in this chapter, the source of the problem of stuttering has remained elusive and obscure for centuries. Learned men in succeeding generations have probed all of the observable and nonobservable signs of the problem and have offered explanations for the occurrence of stuttering.

The search continues for the answers to many questions concerning stuttering. The primary questions that need to be answered are as follows:

1. What causes stuttering initially?
2. Why does stuttering have its onset in childhood between the ages of two and four years?
3. Why do some children become relieved of the problem of stuttering by the age of five or six years?
4. Why do some children continue to stutter through adolescence into adult life and never realize ameliorization of the problem?
5. Why is there a complex of symptoms associated with stuttering?
6. Why do these symptoms vary from person to person?
7. Why does stuttering behavior fluctuate from situation to situation?
8. Why does stuttering defy correction?

It is this author's opinion that these are the most important questions requiring answers if the problem of stuttering is to be understood and more normal speech made possible.

The problem of stuttering has been one of the primary interests of the author for over a quarter of a century. Exploration and study have been ongoing during this period of time, with a relentless search for some of the answers to the foregoing questions. Many blind avenues have been searched to no avail. Theories advanced by others have been reviewed and discarded because they did not satisfactorily answer all of the questions.

The author's speech and language background has been neurologically based. Throughout his college years and up to the present time, emphasis has been placed on studying any and all subject matter that might contribute to a better understanding of the science of speech and language based on neurological and related areas. Other fields of study have included psychology, neuropsychology, educational psychology, neuroanatomy, anatomy, and kinesiology. Through many of these years, the author has been deeply indebted to three learned scholars and notable contributors to the field of speech and language science for their assistance, direction, guidance, and teaching: Martin F. Palmer, Sci.D.; Temple Fay, M.D., and Clarence Simon, Ph.D., all now deceased.

With the foregoing background and years of exploration and experience, the author has found a possible answer for each of the eight primary questions previously advanced.

The basic cause of stuttering appears to be neurophysiological. Research on specific areas of the nervous system during the past few years has revealed some probable areas that could be directly involved in the initiation of the problem. For years this author has searched for a clearer understanding of how motor behaviors of human beings are learned, stored, recalled, and used in consistent pattern form. The answers received or gathered were unsatisfactory or insufficient; there had to be something else. Recent exploration of the functions of the cerebellum, the neocerebellum in particular, began to provide some definitive answers.

The neocerebellum now has been found to be responsible for almost all voluntary motor muscle behavior patterns of human beings. It stores these learned patterns. When an individual needs a specific behavior, the request is directed by way of the cerebral cortex to the cerebellum, where it is programmed. A computed resultant of the program is transmitted to the cerebral motor strip, which then initiates the muscle behaviors necessary to carry out the program.

The author's theory holds that the cause of stuttering is directly related to cerebellar function between the ages of two and four years. This function is normal; there are no problems in the nervous system. Thus, the onset of stuttering is a normal developmental phenomenon. The problem is remediated as the nervous system grows, matures, and becomes increasingly myelinated.

During the period of normal nonfluency, because of conditions beyond his control, the person who continues to stutter changes his thought-to-speech behavior so that now he is not thinking or speaking as a fluent speaker. Only a small percentage of children are victims of this change. They now learn to think and speak in an entirely different sequence that brings about a neurophysiological aberration, which results in the continuation of the stuttering behavior.

As the problem progresses, there are changes in all of the behaviors that constitute oral communication. The individual also strives to do all that he can to eliminate the tonic and clonic blocks in his speech. He tries to accomplish this elimination by resorting to a wide variety of motor acts in order to distract himself from his disabling thought-to-speech patterns. He is unaware of all of the physical and mental activities that are occurring. He is unaware of his different thinking behaviors. The distractions soon lose their effectiveness and become permanent secondary symptoms. All of these behaviors tend to accumulate and form a symptom complex resulting in the syndrome of stuttering.

Efforts directed toward the remediation of stuttering would appear to need to encompass therapeutic procedures for the elimination or correction of all of the symptoms of the complex. Programs designed to bring about the remission of this or that symptom, whichever it may be, are not sufficient for a total correction of the problem. Complete rehabilitative methods will need to be scheduled in a systematic sequence so that each step will lead progressively to the ultimate goal of more normal fluent speech and a complete change in thought-to-speech behavior.

A therapy program that may aid many individuals who stutter is suggested later in this book. Perhaps it will assist them in realizing more fluent speaking behaviors.

Summary

This chapter has opened a discussion of the problem of stuttering and the many questions and possible answers that have been ongoing for centuries. The problem has attracted the concern of many intelligent individuals. Considerable effort and money have been expended in attempting to resolve the mysteries of this disheartening speech disorder. Perhaps there is truly an all-encompassing answer, or it may be that each person who has nonfluent speech is an entity unto himself and that each enigma will need to be resolved on an individual basis. This seems to be rather unlikely in that there are too many common symptoms from person to person.

What actually causes stuttering may never be known. There is, however, always the possibility that someone may stumble onto the true cause of stuttering and the reasons for its continuation throughout life. It is not intended that this writing be the total answer to the problem. It is the desire of the author to stimulate thinking along new lines of reasoning and facilitate new research and experimentation that will eventually result in finding the correct answers to the problem of stuttering. May this manuscript initiate such a desire in the reader.

Chapter 2

PREVAILING THEORIES

IT IS A DIFFICULT and exhausting task to review all of the existing literature available concerning the problem of stuttering. It is by necessity that a selection has been made, and those authors who have been the most quoted and appear to be widely recognized for their contributions will be recognized.

Authorities who are held in high regard during this modern era have had many predecessors dating as far back in history as the Egyptians. There has been considerable redundancy in the thinking of those who have attempted to solve the riddle of stuttering and resolve the problems of those afflicted by this demoralizing speech handicap.

Theories of note tend to fall into three categories, namely (1) stuttering as a learned behavior; (2) stuttering as the result of a psychoneurotic or psychological conflict; and (3) stuttering as the result of a neurological or physiological variation.

STUTTERING AS A LEARNED BEHAVIOR

The most ardent advocate and widely known of the authorities who have promoted the philosophy that stuttering is a learned behavior was Wendell Johnson. [Johnson (1942) termed his deduction the "Diagnosogenic Theory." He stressed that stuttering develops after someone makes the diagnosis that it is happening and not before.] This diagnosis is usually made by laymen, most likely the parents of the child. Their labeling, their reactions, and their attitudes are toward, or of, those normal hesitations that are so characteristic of most young children's speech. Johnson stated that "a child who has been labeled as a

14

stutterer is likely to reflect on this evaluation of his speech and exert considerable effort to avoid nonfluencies." Thus, normal children learn to "develop a hesitation to hesitate."

It would appear that Johnson suggested that children learn to stutter because they are labeled as stutterers. This seems to occur in an environment where the parents are perfectionistic, overanxious, and have an exaggerated concern for their child's welfare. If the parents have had an affiliation with someone who stutters, or have knowledge of the problem of stuttering, they tend to have an amplified reaction to their child's nonfluent speech.

There are many in the field of speech pathology who have been attracted to Johnson's theory, and considerable follow-up research has been done by those who share his ideas.

Oliver Bloodstein (1958) has related to portions of Johnson's theory in his concept of stuttering as an "anticipatory struggle reaction." He was concerned with the conditions under which children began to exhibit strenuous blocks and struggle reactions in their speech. He introduced two factors for consideration. One was the amount of hesitancy a child exhibits, and the other, from Johnson, was concerned with the degree of tolerance the parents had with this hesitant speech.

Bloodstein reflected that there are high standards for fluent speech and behavior in certain segments of our socioeconomic structure. Parents insist on these high standards because of the competition in their social groups. Children who stutter tend to have parents who are more exacting in their child-training policies.

Bloodstein placed considerable importance on fluency and nonfluency. He emphasized the circumstances of certain environmental influences on the child's speech. References were made to the frequent competition with others for an opportunity to speak, the need to verbalize new and exciting experiences, and the necessity to communicate under conditions that are emotionally charged. His assumption is that, no matter what the form or the cause of the nonfluency, any tendency toward nonfluency in an environment reflecting strong disapproval toward the nonfluency will tend to result in habitual anticipatory struggle reactions.

Bloodstein subdivided the development of stuttering into a number of phases. He stressed that all stutterers do not pass through all the stages. There are some young stutterers who develop some of the severe phases of the problem.

In phase one Bloodstein placed the preschool and younger school child whose speech is marked with repetitions of sounds, syllables, and small words at the beginning of a phrase. Prolongations and blocks may be severe but are not common. The child's speech behavior varies with some periods of fluency. The problem becomes worse when the child is placed in speaking situations that may be stressful. There are no secondary symptoms.

In phase two he placed the school child who is a little older and whose problem has become chronic. At this level, speech is marked with repetitions, prolongations, and blocking; hard contacts and blocking are more prevalent. Secondary symptoms are developing. The child recognizes that he is a stutterer but shows no embarrassment or avoidance talk.

The symptoms of the problem have continued to develop in phase three. The occurrence of repetitions has declined, but there has been a continuation of hard blocks and contacts. Secondary symptoms have been elaborated by way of sound and word difficulties, word substitutions, and situational difficulties. The stutterer shows little avoidance or emotional reaction to his speech and continues to talk freely.

All fully developed adult and adolescent stutterers are placed in phase four. The individual now has a severe speech disorder and reflects an emotional reaction to his problem. He anticipates difficulties with words and situations. His use of word substitutions is common and progressively debilitating. Life is not normal because of his avoidance of difficult speaking situations. The stutterer develops a defeatist attitude and becomes preoccupied with his speech problem.

Bloodstein has summed up his theory by stating that "stuttering occurs as the result of the child's conscientious effort to speak acceptably despite a deep conviction that he cannot do so." The problem has its onset during the development of language when speech failures are frequent. Girls are ahead of boys in this activity, so fewer of them develop stuttering. Stuttering reflects a society that "promotes intense competition for status and prestige, and capriciously accepts the most trivial refinements of speech as valid symbols of their attainment."

Wischner (1950), in his treatise, presented a theoretical analysis of stuttering in which he theorized that stuttering behavior is learned, and the motivational component in stuttering is anxiety or anxiety drive. Stuttering behavior involves a learned anxiety reaction system. He compared this anxiety system to those learned in certain kinds of conditioning and learning experiments based on noxious stimuli designed to facilitate an avoidance reaction. The organism learns to avoid noxious stimulation by reacting appropriately to a signal (conditioned stimulus) that occurs prior to the noxious stimulation. An avoidance reaction seems to correlate with expectancy or anxiety. The occurrence or nonoccurrence of stuttering appears to be correlated with the presence or absence of anxiety.

For Wischner, the development of anxiety in a child is caused by the disapproval and censuring of his nonfluent speech by adults in his environment; parents and teachers. Because of these reactions by the adults, the child develops painful reactions that become response-produced stimulation, which evokes anxiety. The child is driven to activities designed to avoid the noxious stimulation. The stimulus cues present include persons and words, cues that instigate anxiety in the adult stutterer.

Wischner stated that there are at least two hypotheses concerning the relationship between anxiety and stuttering. The first one assumes that, although anxiety is learned, stuttering is not learned, but is a disorganized speech behavior caused by the state of anxiety that involves the speech act. His second hypothesis assumes that both anxiety and stuttering are learned.

To support his hypotheses, Wischner referred to two of Mowrer's assumptions. First, he stated that, when anticipatory tensions are intense and not diminished by the reactions they produce, no learning may take place, and there may be a disintegra-tion of behavior. His second reference was that the anxiety is a drive state, which motivates behavior that leads to an escape from a painful stimulation. He related this to stuttering by stating that the child may avoid disapproval (painful stimulation) by not talking at all, or the pressure to communicate may be so great that a conflict develops between the desire to talk and the fear of talking in a certain way. The child may then try to speak in a number of different ways. The pattern of speech used most often will be that which is not followed by punish-ment or disapproval. In spite of the disapproval, the child may continue to speak with nonfluencies because it was these faulty habits that originally initiated the anxiety-producing series of events.

Wischner then related five mechanisms that perpetuate stut-tering behavior. Stuttering may be reinforced by —

1. Virtue of its relatively close association with anxiety-tension re-duction accompanying the removal of a feared word.
2. The anxiety reduction accompanying the escape from a feared situation.
3. The tension reduction consequent upon the completion of a stuttered word.
4. Numerous secondary gains connected with stuttering behavior.
5. A self-verification by the stutterer of his expectation of stutter-ing.

Wischner considered a sixth possibility for the perpetuation of stuttering based on laboratory experiments. The extinction of responses set up by avoidance conditioning is relatively dif-ficult. The elimination of such responses can occur only if there is no response to the danger signal followed by the discovery that there has been no noxious stimulus.

Stutterers may consciously use certain facial and bodily move-ments because they feel such movements help them get the word out. Wischner proposed that these movements become inte-grated into the total stuttering pattern through continual rein-forcement.

For Wischner, then, stuttering behavior is a learned anxiety reaction system to words, situations, and persons.

Many other investigators have supported the learning theory as the cause of stuttering, but these authors appear to have laid the groundwork for most other philosophies.

STUTTERING AS A RESULT OF PSYCHONEUROTIC OR PSYCHOLOGICAL CONFLICT

The proponents of the psychoneurotic and psychological theories of stuttering appear to be at extremes as concerns their thinking. The psychoanalyst leans heavily on Freudian psychology.

In general, psychoanalysts regard stuttering as a neurotic disorder in which a personality disorder is in part reflected in the disturbance of speech. It is held that stuttering results from a struggle to prevent certain thought patterns from emerging as speech that is unacceptable, unrealistic, and instinctual in meaning. Speech is the concrete action of instincts before they are tamed as an ego function. Speech is an exposure of the self acting out instinctual drives. Vocalizing may represent the id, or the id being served by the primitive ego. Utterances may express an attack or desire to be attacked in an oral, phallic, or anal manner. They may indicate a wish to exhibit one's self, to be a voyeur, or a wish to be hurt, to get masochistic pleasure, to be loved, or to be reprimanded. The urge to talk may represent all of these components of the unconscious mind.

Psychoanalytic theory has stated that stuttering is the result of the aforementioned aspects of the ego-id conflict. The ego has to defend itself against the threatening expressions of the id (instincts), which endangers the self and others.

Glauber (1958) stated that his interest in stuttering related to its differentiated aspects and used structural and economic orientations as well as aggressive drive. He delved into the genetic aspects. He reflected that the problem is generally accepted as a pregenital conversion or a narcissistic neurosis, one in which the ego, the executive organ of the reality principle, is defective or insufficiently developed.

According to Glauber, pregenital conversion is the failure of the ego to mature, a fixation at an early ego state. The fixation is manifested in the total personality and speech. The speech symptoms represent an attempt, and an unsuccessful one, to bind the underlying anxiety. With the stutterer, when speech is impending in social situations, anxiety is aroused because of the danger of the assertion of an early ego state, the id, upon the current ego state, where sublimation results in conforming to the demands of society.

Glauber related to two phenomena in stuttering: fixation and regression. Fixation appears to be the result of an interference or the "symbolic function of the ego," or of the oral apparatus becoming involved with other instinctual zones: anal and phallic. When a stutterer is supposed to speak, he may unconsciously want to bite or suck. Thus, a conflict occurs between some elements of biting or sucking and the attempts to block these expressions by forgetting, being quiet, and/or stuttering. According to Glauber, oral fixation is "the key factor in the neurogenesis of stuttering."

There are other theorists who have regarded stuttering as a symptom of psychoneurotic conflict. According to the *Psychiatric Dictionary* (1971), ". . . stuttering is regarded as due in most instances to displacement of anal libido onto the throat and mouth and onto the act of word-forming." The anal-sadistic stutterer equates words with feces. The expulsion or retention of words means the initiation or restriction of anal activity. Words acquire the some omnipotence they had in the infantile stage: "Words can kill." The stutterer is constantly anxious about using such dangerous weapons. While anal sadism forms the core of the problem, other elementary instincts contribute to the symptom. Phallic impulses, for example, may be equated with potency and the ability to speak, and castration with the inability to express oneself. "Whether originating as a physiological disorder or not, in its subsequent states, stuttering is predominantly a psychic condition where there is shrinking from speaking because of the fear of not succeeding."

Stein (1953) believed that stutterers have an infantile personality organization that renders them vulnerable to intrapsychic anxiety. Their response to this anxiety is by way of a regression to an autoerotic rhythmic repetition of sounds and words similar to infant babbling. As stuttering further develops, this infantile erotic speech is accompanied by prolongations as expressions of aggressions, and glottal stops that are regarded as primitive reactions to anxiety. According to Stein, this gratification of infantile needs by stuttering means it is not a conversion but a compulsion neurosis.

Kanner (1957) stated that stuttering is the child's reaction to emotional stress. The child from three to five years old is developing physiological control of the habits of excretion, feeding, sleeping, and speaking. Anxiety at this time, whether it arises from within the child or from the child's relationship with his parents or environment, often finds expression as a disturbance in the maturation of these basic habits. With increasing age and emotional maturity, either the problem giving rise to the anxiety is resolved, or the child establishes control over these functions despite the continuance of the anxiety. These developmental disorders decline and disappear with the passage of time. Kanner suggested that in some young children there is good evidence that stuttering follows this pattern. In some children, while the other problems decrease, stuttering tends to persist and develop further.

Barbara (1962) has written that stuttering may occur in emotionally vulnerable children. This may be caused by a variety of factors resulting where social situations take on new and disturbing significance. The child becomes different from other children as soon as the stuttering occurs and secondary elaborations of neurotic manifestations related to his speech appear. This results in two basic problems: a primary intrapsychic neurotic conflict that renders the child vulnerable, and a secondary elaboration of symptoms as the child, handicapped both by emotional difficulty and speech disorder, tries to communicate his needs and wants. He clings to an idealized image of himself as not handicapped, as a protective compensation. In spite of this he vacillates between being committed to speaking situations in which he will fail and avoiding important ones in which he would probably succeed. For Barbara, this is neurotic behavior.

A theory not related to neurotic behavior but based primarily on psychological implications was proposed by Sheehan (1953). He considered stutterers to be "speech doubters" who are caught in a conflict between wanting to speak and fearing to speak. The conflict, making use of the learning theory of Dollard and Miller, is an approach-avoidance conflict.

Sheehan established two propositions to account for the momentary block in speech and the subsequent release from the block. The conflict hypothesis holds that the stutterer stops speaking whenever conflicting approach-avoidance tendencies reach a state of balance. The fear-reduction aspects of this theory state that the occurrence of the stuttering reduces the fear that caused it, so that during the block there is sufficient reduction in the fear-motivated avoidance to resolve the conflict and thus permit the release of the blocked word.

Sheehan noted that a stutterer has two alternatives, to speak or to remain silent. While speaking achieves communication, it also brings shame and guilt because of the stuttering. To remain silent results in no stuttering, but is also followed by shame and guilt for not communicating. The conflict between these alternatives, when each has positive and negative components, is best viewed as a double approach-avoidance conflict. When these conflicting drives approach a stalemate, there will tend to be an oscillation about this point as first one and then the other becomes predominant. It is this oscillation that produces the principal stuttering symptoms of repetition and prolongation. Secondary symptoms are considered to be either compensatory acts to overcome the stuttering blocks, or the stutterer's conscious attitude toward the listener.

Sheehan suggested that it is profitable to consider approach-avoidance conflicts at five distinct levels:

1. At the word level, through past conditioning on that particular word. This is directly comparable to Wischner's specific word anxiety.

2. On the situation level, when learning in previous speech situations results in an unwillingness to enter them again. This is comparable to general situation anxiety.

3. When there is conflict due to the emotional content of speech. He cited as evidence the increase in stuttering when personally derogatory material is used.

4. When there is conflict on an interpersonal relationship level: for instance, the common increase in stuttering when speaking to authority figures.

5. On an ego-protective level, stuttering serves unconsciously as a means of keeping the individual out of competitive endeavors that would pose a threat of failure or a threat of success.

Sheehan also related to guilt as a source of conflict in stuttering. Both primary and secondary guilt are found and secondary guilt is far more significant. Primary guilt relates to the feelings behind the onset of the stuttering. Secondary guilt is the reaction the stutterer develops through his thinking that his blocks are distressing to others. Guilt feelings may be in the background of the onset of stuttering. In the adult and the young secondary stutterer, guilt seems to result from the role playing that becomes a part of the stutterer's behavior.

He stated that, in the later stages of treatment, the relationship of fluency to guilt becomes more apparent because the stutterer believes that, since his fluencies are false, he is undeserving of honest fluency.

The preceding authorities have determined that the precipitating factors in stuttering are psychoneurotic and/or psychological. They have based their thinking on observations of those behaviors that lend themselves to the principles of these two philosophies.

STUTTERING AS THE RESULT OF A NEUROLOGICAL OR PHYSIOLOGICAL VARIATION

Many investigators have explored a wide realm of possible neurological and physiological causes for stuttering. It will be noted that, while some have suggested such an etiology, they also have incorporated some psychological considerations.

Berry (1956) offered the observation that there is an increase in the incidence of encephalitis or epilepsy in the stuttering population.

MacKeith and Bax (1962) suggested that perhaps there was a minimal structural change in the central nervous system of these persons.

West (1968) has postulated that stuttering is a variant of epilepsy. He had stated his hypothesis earlier (1958): "Stuttering is primarily an epileptic disorder that manifests itself in dyssynergies of the neuromotor mechanism for oral language." He continued by saying that the "spasms" were caused by social anxieties associated with communication. Such anxieties are the result of moral training and precipitate stuttering when they take on "the form of conscious feelings of guilt." This is enhanced if the guilt concerns what the individual says and how he says it.

West related primary stuttering to a convulsive disorder and involved a certain relationship to those around the stutterer. The phenomenon does not occur outside communication and social interactions. He found that this was the primary difference between stuttering and petit mal epilepsy.

More recently, West (1968) set forth the theory that stuttering may have three possible causes that may work independently or jointly: (1) "atavistic heredity," (2) "brain injury," and (3) "hysteroid dysfluencies." He noted that it is impossible to know which of these etiologies produces the greatest number of stutterers.

He theorized that stuttering may result from atavistic heredity, remote inheritance, or delayed evolution that prevents the development of a feedback for fluent patterns of oral communication. Some stuttering may be thought of as a failure of the development of speech fluency in the process of human evolution. The relationship of stuttering to twinning, left-handedness, allergies, and vulnerability to respiratory infections may be that those phenomena are related to delayed evolutionary factors.

He continued his theory by saying that some stuttering may be a form of subclinical cerebral palsy. "Certainly it often exhibits itself in known cases of brain damage." He related to his earlier thinking conjoining stuttering and epilepsy, inferring that primary stuttering is a close relative of pyknolepsy.

Departing from his neurological and physiological hypothesizing, West noted that stuttering may be "purely hysterical." The speech characteristics of stuttering may be unconsciously used to gain attention. It may be an "alingering — conscious or otherwise — to get persons out of active military duty, or onto the rolls of the insurance agency."

West has listed five characteristics that classify stuttering as a speech defect. There are breaks in articulate speech and phonation. When such breaks occur, there are facial and bodily tensions that are reactions to frustration and straining to override the breaks and resume the normal flow of speech. Spasms of a tonic or clonic nature appear in the speech musculature during the breaks in speech. One symptom on which he placed special emphasis is the appearance of various "tics" in the muscles of phonation and remote musculature during breaks.

He implied that these characteristics may be taken as a definition of stuttering, but stated that ". . . realistically stuttering is the type of speech used when a speaker and his listener agree that the speaker stutters."

To be sure that what is occurring is actually stuttering, West commented that there must be a differentiation from other forms of speech in which breaks occur, such as Jacksonian epilepsy, petit mal seizures, and certain psychoses. In stuttering, the stutterer is impeded in speech by sudden failures of automatic control. He is caught in a conflict between voluntary control of individual speech movements on the one hand and voluntary initiation of automatic serial responses on the other.

The best criterion to use in differentiating stuttering from other similar speech conditions, according to West, is by noting the appearance of associated "tics." Unfortunately, these tics are not apparent in beginning stuttering. He presented an evolution of the stutterer's tics:

1. The search for some device to help him override or camouflage the stuttering spasm.
2. The discovery of such a device. It may be a moving of the feet along the floor, a frown, a turning of the head, a starting word or

phrase like *so,* or *now,* or *well,* or *I mean to say.*

3. The stereotype or habituation of such a device.

4. The unconscious and automatic use of such a device whenever the patient is impeded in speech. By this time the tic has been so firmly associated with the block that the twain are virtually incorporated into a single psychomotor mechanism.

Thus, for West, the most valid criterion of distinction between stuttering and incidental blocking of speech is the presence or absence of associated tics. Their presence in association with sudden lapses in speech usually signifies stuttering.

Eisenson (1956) inferred that stuttering is a manifestation of perseveration, and that most stutterers are predetermined because they are "constitutionally inclined to perseverate to a greater degree than most speakers." There are a number of persons who stutter because they are confronted with factors and influences that cause them to perseverate at the moment of speaking.

By definition, perserveration is the continuance of an activity after the cessation of the stimulus that caused it. It may appear in clonic form, repeated movement, or tonic form, where a position is maintained (Dorland, 1957).

Therefore, according to Eisenson, when a person who stutters blocks, repeats, prolongs, or has repetitive ticlike behaviors, he is perseverating.

This perseverative behavior takes place in speaking situations whenever the speaker finds himself to be unequal to the task. Perseveration may be either organic or psychological in origin, or a combination of both. If it is organic in nature, it may indicate a "mild amnesic" problem for word finding during various levels of verbal exchange. This may arise because of variations in cortical development. There may be a conflict between cortical and subcortical centers for the control of speech, or there may be cortical tissue damage. The stutterer may function well under ideal conditions in that the degree of neurological difference may be slight.

Eisenson stated that about half of the adolescent and adult stuttering population does not belong to this organic group.

These persons who make up the other half of the stuttering population have learned to stutter by way of imitation and have continued to do so for the psychological rewards or "secondary gain associated with stuttering."

Eisenson added another entity to his stuttering population, namely, "a psychogenic stutterer" whose problem is a result of an early childhood "emotional disturbance." Such stutterers have considerably more difficulty with speech that is not propositional in nature. The psychogenic stutterer will have trouble with things such as series counting and other automatic types of speech responses. It appears that he has trouble if he becomes aware that he will have to initiate the verbal behavior. He seems to be unwilling or unable to separate even meaningless words from himself.

Eisenson, then, emphasized several possible causes for the perseverative phenomenon. The causes he gave consist of "constitutional organic differences, neuropathologies, varying degrees of psychosomatic disturbances and psychopathologies;" in simpler terms, differences in bodily behavior, brain damage, and self-initiated disturbances and psychological problems.

Karlin (1950) is another theorist whose contribution to the cause of stuttering reflects neurological complications. He assumed that there is a delay in the myelinization of the cortical speech areas of the brain, and this is the primary somatic factor that becomes the basis of stuttering. In keeping with this, he reflects on the lower incidence of stuttering in females, noting that they have a greater degree of myelinization during the critical time period of three or four years.

Karlin noted that nerves that have not been completely myelinated may transmit impulses, but the effect may be one of movement lacking in precision and fine coordination. In reference to speech, he stated: "Impulses which are initiated or controlled by a brain cortex that is not well co-ordinated may result in the production of a dysrhythmic, repetitive, interrupted flow of speech."

Karlin noted a secondary factor that may produce stuttering. Psychologically, exposure and reaction of the young child to undue emotional stress and strain during the negativistic period between three and four may cause the problem. However, if the child is managed properly, and if the emotional stress is reduced, the child's speech should improve. This should allow for further myelinization of the brain to take place, permitting the development of the fine coordinated movements for speech.

In his early treatise, Travis (1937) was an exponent of a neurological basis for stuttering. He believed that the specific neurological phenomenon that contributed to stuttering was the tendency for both cerebral hemispheres to be more clearly equal in potential and control of speech functions. He stated that this was not the case in nonstutterers.

Travis (1946) now believes that the neurological variant exists "only as the pathophysiological subsoil of stuttering." The combined effects of a western culture's demand for a renunciation of infantile and childish behavior at an early age and the possession of somatic variant in some of these infants and children produce stuttering. Such children are unsuccessful in their attempts to deal with a given life demand. They are unable to "find socially acceptable gratification of their subjective needs under given circumstances."

Travis thus has believed that a child who becomes a stutterer begins with a deviant cerebral mechanism that prolongs infantile behavior and has a difficult beginning in making adjustments. As he grows older, he does not mature emotionally, but continues to employ infantile adjustment patterns. Early forces of wishes, hates, and fears become part of the stutterer's expression and, therefore, the symptomology of stuttering. Stuttering "may be conceptualized then as the final defense or block against the threatening revelation through spoken words of unspeakable thoughts and feelings."

Schwartz (1976), in his book *Stuttering Solved*, stated that stuttering in the child is directly related to what he calls the "airway dilation reflex." He defined this reflex as "a vigorous dilation of the airway prior to strong inhalation." The nostrils, throat, and vocal cords all dilate during this reflex. Speech requires air pressure. The child's brain misinterprets this increase in air pressure as a life-threatening airway obstruction and triggers off the reflex automatically.

Schwartz believed that the dilation reflex is responsible for stuttering in that, in counteracting this phenomenon, the stutterer closes the vocal cords strongly in laryngospasm. He learns to lock the vocal folds with excessive tension, and this precipitates all of the struggling observed in the young stutterer. As the child matures, the air dilation reflex is outgrown. What is seen in the adult stutterer is a learned stimulus response and is pure habit.

Schwartz also added the stress factor to his theory. He stated that "stress produces the conditioned reflex of the vocal cord tension, which, in turn, produces the conditioned reflex of extricatory struggle behavior, the stuttering." He listed seven main stresses that are involved in stuttering with an additional "baseline stress" that produces tension in all of the muscles of the body at one time. In tying this into his theory, he noted that the vocal cords are extremely sensitive indicators of this kind of stress.

Although Schwartz listed four different kinds of stuttering, he said that his first two types are the most predominant. Type I, diagrammed in his book, basically indicates stress as the initiator, followed by a laryngospasm; then speech occurs with the obvious struggle reaction. Type II also shows stress as the initiating agent, followed by a laryngospasm, but the "obvious struggle" precedes speech output. "Obvious struggle" is the stuttering that occurs in attempting to speak.

Bryngelson (1940) believed that stuttering is an "atavistic state" in which the individuals have "an ambilateral rather than unilateral neurological control over speech." He stated that this is probably due to an arrested development of the neural system.

While there have been many who have considered possible neurological and/or physiological causes for stuttering, this review will note a statement by one more author.

Palmer (1937) was a strong advocate of the theory that stuttering was a phenomenon of neurophysiological origin rather than a so-called volitional or emotional disturbance. In studying the cardiac cycle as a physiological determinant of energy distributions in speech, he found that circulatory rhythms determine the distribution of energy in a definite significant pattern. He also found that stutterers, when speaking, did not follow the tendencies of normal speakers.

Palmer (1951) reported on many neurophysiological differences that were observed between the total speech behaviors of normal speakers and stutterers. He referred to the interesting parallels between certain types of cerebral palsy and stuttering. The parallel to athetosis was noted in particular in that persons with this type of cerebral palsy had speech and related behaviors that looked like those observed in stuttering. The comparisons could be made if the person with athetosis could talk, be placed in the moderately severe group, and if consideration could be localized to the speech organs. Here, it was noted that there were repetitions, hesitations, prolongations, or differentiations in the time values of speech. The spasms, etc., were intermittent. The quiet and speech breathing patterns were deviant. The remainder of the description of the phenomena, excluding sex indexes, could not be distinguished. The emotional status, etc., of the person with athetosis is parallel, item for item, on all things ever seen or said about stutterers. Stuttering and cerebral palsy conditions are not the same. Cerebral palsy is a problem in which there are divergent muscle behaviors as the result of selective damage to the central nervous system.

Stuttering and cerebral palsy are propositional disorders in that the severity of the problem depends on the propositionality of the situation. For example, as the premium placed on a behavior increases, the greater the pressure on the performance. It is so with both of these problems: the more pressure there is exerted for performing, the worse the problems become. The level of propositionality is determined by the person, not by the situation. The individual determines how important or pressurized each event is to him, and this affects his behavior.

Palmer (1939) remarked concerning the differences noted in the breathing patterns of persons who stutter, and those of normal speakers. Not only were there deviations in the speech breathing patterns; there were variations in the quiet breathing patterns. Kymograph recordings and analysis showed that the stutterer's speech breathing patterns were out of phase, irregular, and quite different from those of their normal counterparts. The quiet breathing patterns were also found to be not synchronized, irregular, and shallow when compared to those of normal subjects.

Over the years, Palmer studied the various organic systems and their possible implication in stuttering. Stuttering begins before the age of puberty and is associated with childhood. Although some cases do occur after puberty, this appears to be the magic line. Statistics indicate two peaks for the onset of stuttering: two to four and five to seven years. The second age level tends to be artificial. It is of critical importance that the problem begins at the earlier age. Boy stutterers outnumber the girls three to one. Physiologically, there are differences between the sexes; basically, there are differences in the metabolisms at this age, slight, but there.

Palmer and his medical staff explored the possible involvement of the endocrine system in stuttering and noted that certain drugs affected the endocrine and nervous systems and caused stuttering in some persons.

They found that the heartbeat of the male stutterer was more irregular and rapid than that of normal speakers. Female stutterers were found not to be different from male normals. As female stutterers grow older, their rhythms become more normal and calm. The male stutterer's rhythms tend to stay the same or become worse.

In another study conducted by Palmer and his medical staff, it was found that the incidence of stuttering was nonexistent in a population of over 45,000 individuals who had diabetes. It appeared that persons with diabetes, or those who were to have this problem, did not stutter.

Palmer broached the question whether stutterers were emotionally maladjusted by noting that other types of speech-handicapped individuals displayed the same emotional configurations as stutterers, namely, anxiety and fear. He stated that proof was lacking to say that stuttering was caused by emotional problems. There are many individuals with emotional problems, children included, who do not stutter. Psychological tests do not reveal a specific pattern or profile for stutterers.

Palmer was convinced that there were no gross traumatic lesions causing stuttering. In support of his thinking, he stressed that it was possible to have anatomical dysfunctions with an intact nervous system. Children who should have had gross lesions in the nervous system because of a severe anatomical involvement showed no evidence to support the dysfunction when an autopsy was performed. The source of the problem may have been metabolic.

Palmer explored in detail the mechanics of language and speech as carried out by the nervous system. He noted that, if there was a neurological involvement in stuttering, dysfunction in the thalamo-cortico-stria pathways would be the most likely site. The symptomology of stuttering could be well explained with such an entanglement. He was very much interested in the suppressor circuits in the nervous system and questioned their possible contribution to stuttering. He was concerned with the lack of research in these areas.

Van Riper (1954) held to a theory that stuttering may have many origins. He noted, as have most, that the difficulty usually begins between the ages of two and four years. This is the period when children are normally having some trouble mastering the fluency skills of language. Most children show some fluency during this period. Van Riper believed that these children are exposed to "fluency disruptors" that influence their speech.

He has characterized these disruptors as competition from adults who are superior in their abilities as well as in their authorities and interrupt the child's attempts to vocalize his feelings and thoughts. Many survive this ordeal with little or no effects on their speech. Those who become stutterers are not equal to the pressures and demands placed upon them.

Van Riper believed that children who become stutterers may be distinguished in one of the following ways:

1. They may have low frustration tolerance.

2. They may have speech environments with an excess of fluency disruption.

3. They may have a constitutional predisposition (dysphemia) to prolong nonfluency or to stuttering.

4. They may have parents who misevaluate their speech or for some other reason react to their non-fluencies with anxiety, or penalty, or both.

5. They may be ones for whom dysrhythmic, non-fluent speech may be at manifestation of an underlying emotional conflict.

6. They may be victims of some combination of the above.

He distinguished between normal nonfluency and primary stuttering. He also made a distinction between primary and secondary stuttering. When the stutterer begins to objectify his problem, becomes apprehensive as he approaches situations requiring speech, and scrutinizes words with anxiety, he has become a secondary stutterer. Secondary stutterers tend to self-perpetuate their problems.

The symptoms of stuttering may become reinforced in many ways, one of which is an error in judgment where two sequential bits of behavior are misinterpreted as cause and effect acts. The utterance of the word by the stutterer terminates his distress. He feels that his struggle reaction was responsible for his release from anxiety. To maintain this release from anxiety, the stutterer makes the decision that he must repeat this behavior again and again.

Van Riper believed that the most likely cause of stuttering results from parents labeling their child's normal nonfluencies as abnormal. The child's attempts to talk in phrases and sentences, to please his parents before he is developmentally ready, create anxiety and stress. However it originates, stuttering tends to maintain itself once it does commence.

This author has attempted to present a brief overview of the thinking of the most heralded theorists in the field working with the problem of stuttering. While most of the authors mentioned have varying opinions as to the cause of stuttering, many of them are as one in their thinking as concerns the perpetuation of the problem after the initial phase of primary nonfluencies. To a large extent, they lean heavily on psychological problems or some form of neurotic behavior. They seem to feel that beyond the young primary state of stuttering, one must search for some underlying emotional provocation.

Summary

A review of the most accepted theories to date has been presented to provide the reader needed information to better appraise the new look at the old problem of stuttering. Many have expressed opinions as to the cause of this demoralizing speech handicap to the extent that volumes have been written. Only those authorities or theorists who have gained recognition and prominence have their theories reviewed here. Most other opinions tend to be modifications or embellishments of these major theories.

Authors reviewed include Bloodstein, Bryngelson, Eisenson, Glauber, Johnson, Karlin, Palmer, Schwartz, Sheehan, Travis, Van Riper, West, Wischner, and others. If any authors have been omitted who feel that their theories are sound, this author apologizes; it was impossible to include everyone.

Although there are varying opinions as to the cause of stuttering in the young child, the protraction of the problem into older childhood, adolescence, and adulthood appears to be psychological or psychopathic in nature. This opinion appeared to be unanimous among the majority of the theorists reviewed.

In spite of the large number of theories advanced and held to be reasonably valid, none appears to readily solve the riddle of the cause of stuttering nor of its continuation beyond the primary, young child phase.

Chapter 3

CURRENTLY RECOGNIZED THERAPEUTIC PROCEDURES

OVER THE YEARS that individuals have been stuttering, many concerned investigators have tried to arrive at solutions to the problem that would ameliorate the woes suffered by so tormented a group. Since the beginning of the history of the problem, every conceivable corrective procedure has been advocated. Early remedies included running up hills to improve the breathing, cauterizing the tongue, talking with pebbles in the mouth, and performing acts to purge the devils and evil spirits that existed in these distressed persons.

Those who have advanced a theory as to the cause and protraction of stuttering have also suggested therapies or treatments for the alleviation of the problem. Many treatment programs prescribed today are designed, not so much to alleviate the problem, but to make it more palatable and reduce the severity of the characteristics that are felt to be indicative of the suffering of the person who stutters.

As with most problems, the major emphasis has been directed toward relieving the observable signs of stuttering. While many have listed varying characteristics of stuttering, it is the opinion of this author that most will agree on those to be presented here.

When a person stutters, there is an abnormal interruption in the flow of speech consisting of repetitions, hesitations, prolongations, and stoppages. In the more severe cases the deviant speech patterns are quite noticeable and characteristically involved to the point that they often detract from what the speaker is trying to say. Most individuals who have stuttered for any

35

length of time have developed some secondary symptoms or characteristics such as eye batting, facial grimacing, labial distortions, and variations in body attitudes and configurations. These symptoms may be mild or excessive. Although these behavioral patterns are usually notably observable in older children and adults, they are often seen as well in the young child who stutters.

Not all therapists, but some who offer treatment, agree that the stutterer has developed a great deal of tension throughout his anatomy, particularly in the musculature used for speaking, and that it is apparent when he is trying to talk.

The tendency of a stutterer to speak with varying degrees of difficulty or fluency is influenced by the circumstances and the situations in which he must communicate. The higher the premium he places on a given speaking encounter, the more difficulty he will experience.

Some authorities believe that the stutterer has some difficulties with and variations in his breathing patterns and that this may be one of the major problems of concern. Some stutterers seem to have to fight for breath and may have problems coordinating laryngeal valving and breathing for speech.

There are those who are of the opinion that the stutterer creates his own difficulties because of his attitude toward his problem and that this is reflected in what he does when he speaks.

Most authorities will agree that there are fluency and nonfluency patterns in the speech of children who stutter. There are periods when a child's speech will be relatively free from the behavioral patterns of stuttering. The tendency for these periods to occur gradually diminishes until, by the time the stutterer reaches adolescence, the probability of a fluent period of speech may be nonexistent.

Stutterers tend to develop anticipatory behaviors. Most adolescent and adult stutterers acquire the inclination to foretell or foresee words or sounds with which they will have difficulty. These individuals will at times resort to substituting another word for the difficult one. More often they do not, and then stuttering occurs on some aspect of that word. There is a tendency for this behavior to be consistent with particular phonemes or words in a given stutterer. It is not uncommon to hear such persons say that they have particular difficulty with the *W*, the *B*, or other specific speech sounds.

With but a few exceptions, the authors reviewed in Chapter 2 of this book indicated that stutterers were victims of some kind of emotional reaction. It was either stated or implied that anxiety was involved to one degree or another.

Anxiety, according to the *Psychiatric Dictionary* (1971), consists of somatic, physiological, and psychological types. Characteristics of the first two types are disturbed breathing, increased heart activity, vasomotor changes, and musculoskeletal disturbances. In the psychological type, there is an inner attitude and feeling characterized by a physical and mental awareness of being powerless to do anything about a personal matter, a presentiment of inevitable danger, a self-absorption that interferes with effective solutions to problems of reality, and doubt concerning the nature of the threatening evil. Anxiety is differentiated from fear in that fear is a reaction to a real or threatened danger. Stutterers are victims of anxiety to the extent that many of these signs are observable to both the trained and the untrained observer.

Not mentioned directly by most, but an obvious result of anxiety, is the probability of stress suffered by those who stutter. Stress is defined as an interference that disturbs the organism's functioning at any level, producing a situation that is natural to avoid, the effect of which is influenced by the meaning of the stress-stimulus to the person. Many stutterers describe feelings, both psychological and physiological, that occur while in certain speaking situations that are characteristic of anxiety and stress.

There are those who will undoubtedly reflect that there are other characteristics of this problem, which should have been mentioned above. The symptoms noted are those most frequently listed as acceptable signs of stuttering. They are mentioned in terms used by other authors.

As stated earlier, most treatment programs have been designed to reduce the severity of the characteristics of stuttering, with a few proclaiming a cure or correction of the problem itself.

Most of the emphasis in the treatment of stuttering has been directed toward the alleviation or eradication of the repetitions, hesitations, prolongations, and stoppages that are paramount in the speech of the stutterer.

One of the quickest and most widely used methods devised to eliminate the speaking characteristics of the stutterer is by way of distractions. This is an age-old procedure and has been effective in the temporary remission of the problem. This course of action involves providing the stutterer with either a motor behavior or a thought process that causes him to be distracted from his manner of speaking. It affords him something to do or think about while he is talking so that he does not think about his speech or about the situation in which he is speaking.

An example of this procedure would be to have the stutterer tap his foot, or wiggle his finger, or describe a figure with his finger or hand while talking. These would be classified as motor distractions. An example of thought distraction would be to have the stutterer concentrate on one particular aspect of his speech to the extent that it alone becomes the focal point of his attention during the process of speaking. Points of concentration could be breathing, laryngeal valving or phonation, or manner of articulation. Other distractions that have been used are role playing, assuming the personality or manner of speaking of someone else, exaggerating the articulation of the phonemes of speech, and overdoing the movements of the lips, tongue, and jaw while articulating the speech sounds. There are many other distractions that would fall into either one or the other of the two categories, motor and thought. The major effect of a distraction is that it takes the stutterer's attention away from the speaking processes and/or situation of the moment, thus allowing his speech to be more fluent.

While this procedure affords the stutterer some temporary relief, there is strong opposition to its use. A distraction is only a temporary trick that serves the stutterer for a short period of time, until it loses its distracting effect. A distraction often becomes a segment of his secondary behaviors.

There are many who propose psychoanalytic therapy for stuttering in that they view the problem as a narcissistic neurosis (Glauber, 1958). The term *psychoanalysis* or *psychoanalytic* can take on several meanings. It seems to apply to the sense of basic science of human behavior and motivation at one extreme and to classical psychoanalysis at the other. The point of concern, which appears to be in the person and in the therapy, is the phobic avoidance or the anticipatory anxiety of speaking situations. This is the difficulty that must be faced from the beginning. A problem arises in the administering of this form of therapy in that the child does not meet the maturity prerequisite for its utilization. Certain requirements, such as age of the patient, motivation, capacity for making use of the therapy as an active experience, and the ability to relinquish secondary gains from the symptom, preclude the use of this therapy for children.

In view of these requirements for actual psychotherapy, adaptations have been advocated for children. Some of the plans advanced are to give only the mother psychoanalysis or psychotherapy, to provide the mother with this treatment while the child receives psychotherapy at the same time, or to provide both mother and child with the full treatment simultaneously.

Here, the mother of the stutterer is drawn to the center of the therapy because of the feeling that in seeking help for her child she is really seeking help for herself. It is suggested that the mother has suffered two severe reactivations of her early separation anxieties, her marriage and the birth of her child. The separation of child from mother freed the child and promoted the growth of his ego. It is suggested that the indirect treatment of the child who stutters is more efficacious than direct therapy because it deals with the basic pathogenesis of the problem.

For the less psychoanalytically oriented and those who are of a psychological view, there appear to be progressive psychotherapeutic procedures that are advised. A major emphasis is placed on reducing the fear of the consequences of stuttering, which can be accomplished only after there is some reduction of the stutterer's emotionalized desire to keep from stuttering.

Some state that the stutterer must learn to speak about his stuttering freely and frankly to others. He must admit his problem to those who may not be aware of it. He should be able to discuss it in difficult and feared situations. He should be able to make an appropriate remark to help him pass off his stuttering lightly in situations where he has difficulty speaking.

There is a growing trend in speech therapy to use a specialized form of psychotherapy. This emphasis is toward group therapy and requires the stutterer to overcome his avoidance of stuttering. Therapy is directed toward helping the stutterer rediscover his stuttering. He should become more aware of listening reactions and note how the listener reacts to his stuttering. Avoidance tendencies, in terms of words and situations, should be reduced. Attempts should be made to break up the relationship between anxiety and stuttering, guilt and stuttering, guilt and silence, and guilt and fluency. Efforts then center on building secure authority relationships.

Some work is being directed toward having the stutterer adopt a new role, that of being a thoroughly integrated and self-accepting stutterer. He must be willing to relinquish the secondary gains realized from his problems. He cannot continue to use stuttering to escape from society or to avoid the threat of failure. By doing this, the stuttering loses any real protective function it may have had.

For the child stutterer, because of his lack of well-developed awareness of the problem and the absence of secondary symptoms, the problem is approached in terms of the general methods of child psychology. Help may be afforded children by way of their parents, through activity therapy or play therapy, or some form of release therapy. Relationship therapy, which deals with varying levels of approach-avoidance and relationship conflicts, is also advocated.

In the treatment of adolescents and adults, hypnosis has been used as a technique for reducing the severity of stuttering. This procedure has been used to supplement other therapies, or for the remission of stuttering by posthypnotic suggestion.

A different form of psychological intervention was suggested by Dunlap (1932). He recommended negative practice by which the stutterer was to practice his own stuttering to the extent that he became aware of the problem and learned to control it.

Bryngelson (1940) encouraged a form of negative practice with voluntary stuttering. The stutterer was to see himself and his speech problem objectively. Each one was to stutter voluntarily when he felt he might encounter nonfluency. The goal was to help the stutterer face speaking situations rather than to avoid them.

Johnson (1939) recommended a program of voluntary stuttering by way of easy repetitions. The therapy was designed to help the stutterer develop control over his stuttering behavior, reduce his tension, and give him a choice of how he wanted to stutter. His intent was to give the stutterer a manner of performing his stuttering more and more simply and easily.

There are many authorities who relate their premises concerning stuttering as being organic or neurogenic in origin yet hold that any relationship between therapist and client is part psychotherapeutic and that all patients need some degree of psychotherapy. The amount and degree of such therapy depends on the individual.

Eisenson (1958) stated that, in dealing with the constitutional perseverator (organic stutterer), therapeutic approaches should be directed toward four objectives. The stutterer must accept himself as a functioning organism. Nonorganic causes that increase the attitudes associated with psychogenic perseveration must be weakened. Stuttering blocks and secondary symptoms must be modified, controlled, and eliminated if possible. The stutterer should speak in conformity with his constitutional predisposition, modify his rate, and speak so that the effort is without the characteristics of stuttering.

Eisenson theorized that, in the constitutional (organic) stutterer, the repetitions and hesitations constitute perseveration. With the inclusion of anxiety, apprehension, and struggle, there is a transformation into stuttering. He emphasized the need for objective evaluation and acceptance of the amount of perseverative oral language the stutterer seems to require in specific situations and the type of situations. Through his approach, he has helped the stutterer to "accept himself for what he cannot help being rather than to be somebody he is constitutionally unable to become."

He further noted that symptomatic treatment and psychotherapy help to weaken the nonorganic causes of stuttering. This, in turn, reduces the nonorganic perseverative reinforcement of the organic cause of the problem and results in a marked decrease in repetitions and hesitations, with speech beginning to approximate the normal.

Van Riper, in *Stuttering: A Symposium* (Eisenson, 1958), outlined his therapy from 1936 to 1957. His early rationale for treatment was as follows:

> 1. Stuttering consists largely of learned behavior which can be modified and reduced through training procedures.
> 2. Stuttering consists largely of avoidance and frustration responses, both of which reinforce stuttering.
> 3. The stutterer's self-concept can be altered so that less stuttering occurs.

Over the years, Van Riper has used a variety of techniques to improve the fate of the stutterers with whom he has worked. At one time, psychotherapy was emphasized and found to be disappointing. Then, the emphasis of the therapy was directed toward speech therapy for the stutterer, with an emphasis on self-therapy.

In self-therapy, stutterers were assigned structured experiences they were to have on a daily basis. These experiences were to be in the following areas: desensitization, nonreinforcement, ego-building, highly conscious voluntary control of the speaking apparatus, self-understanding and exploration, and fluent stuttering.

Van Riper's criteria for successful stuttering therapy, besides being a better speaker than himself, was that the stutterer must not avoid words or speaking situations; his stuttering must not be a deterrent to social or vocational adjustments; his fear of words and situations must be zero; and his stuttering must present no concern to himself or others.

Recently, March, 1978, there has been an increase in the promotion of self-help for stutterers. This approach has been initiated for most of the million or more stutterers in the United States and was stressed in the most recent publication of the Speech Foundation of America (March, 1978). The major emphasis of this therapeutic procedure follows closely the ideas offered by some of the authorities previously mentioned in this chapter, with many suggestions from Van Riper.

Not too many years ago, it was suggested by Cherry et al. (1956) that stuttering might be related to a delay in the auditory feedback loop, or a delay in the stutterer hearing his own speech. There was an attempt to use this method as a therapeutic procedure. A program was developed at the University of Chicago by Goldiamond (1974) whereby stutterers were exposed to delayed auditory feedback as part of their therapy. The developer of this program suggested that it did not eliminate the stuttering, but taught the stutterer new speech patterns. To this author's knowledge, no follow-up reports have been published as to the results of the program or as to the lasting effects of the treatment.

The department of speech of the Bridgeport, Connecticut, Easter Seal Rehabilitation Center was given a wire release of a story concerning their program, which they say brings about the correction of stuttering within nine to twelve hours (UPI, 1977). According to the release and the program developer, Van Kirk, the child was scolded for stuttering and told that "he can't do it anymore." When the child had a problem with a particular word, he was instructed to say the word slowly until he could pronounce it properly without stuttering. When this was accomplished, he was encouraged to say the word faster and faster. The center also suggested that adult stutterers had been corrected in this manner. This approach appears to be based on adaptation to specific word anxiety. How long the remission of stuttering lasts was not disclosed.

Schwartz (1976), in his book, *Stuttering Solved,* stated that his is the first proposal offering a solution to the problem of stuttering. The cause, as noted in Chapter 2, was said to be physical, and his therapy was reportedly successful with a high percentage of patients.

The basis of this treatment recommended by Schwartz is referred to as the "airflow technique." It appears that the stutterer is asked to produce a long, audible sigh. Halfway through the sigh he is asked to say one syllable. The number of syllables per breath is then increased. The person is later asked to make the sigh inaudible. The results are that there is no stuttering.

Schwartz has cautioned that there are five misuses of the airflow, all brought about by one of the seven basic stresses he has listed.

In spite of the success of the airflow method, Schwartz found that stuttering blocks occasionally occurred on the initial sound of the syllable to be spoken. To eliminate this problem, the stutterer was forced to pronounce slowly the first syllable after the start of each flow of air. This again aborted the stuttering.

Schwartz's concern over relapse is summed up in his statement that the patients learned to stutter and they have to "learn their way out of the problem." A total cure would probably take years. The individuals must alter their self-concepts and develop the airflow until it becomes a habit.

There are some conflicting views concerning the use of relaxation as a therapeutic procedure for stuttering. Luper (1978) suggested that stuttering results when the speaker is unable to cope with excessive muscle tension in the speech mechanism. It is suggested that fear and tension are stutterer's greatest enemies. The import is that, if the stutterer had little or no tension, he probably would not stutter or would, at least, stutter more easily. There would be a world of difference if the stutterer could just eliminate his tensions through relaxation.

Self-Therapy for the Stutterer (1978) indicated that relaxation procedures do sometimes produce fluency, but unfortunately, it has been found that they usually have little or no carryover effect. This does not mean that relaxation measures are discouraged since learning to relax cannot help but be of benefit to general health and well-being. According to Gregory (1978), relaxing procedures are not indicated as a solution to stuttering.

It has been advised that, if the stutterer can locate where there is the most tension, it is possible to learn to relax those muscles during speech. Differential muscle exercises are said to be helpful under special circumstances. Relaxation should just involve the muscles used to control the lips, tongue and mouth, breathing, and to some extent, the vocal cords in the throat. This author's concepts concerning relaxation and its effects on stuttering will be explained later.

For a period of time there were those who, because of the theory relating stuttering to the lack of development of true cerebral dominance (Travis, 1937), proposed that a child's handedness be examined and then be changed if indicated. If it was found that there were problems relating to a dominant hand, eye, and foot, it was strongly recommended that the handedness be changed. It was held that this would greatly help to alleviate the problem of stuttering and assist in the establishment of better cerebral dominance.

Another procedure that has been suggested to encourage stutterers to speak fluently has been choral reading. With this therapy the stutterer is to read along with the therapist, and the twoness of the speaking situation and the lowering of the pressure during reading facilitate smooth, noninterrupted speech. It is desired that the stutterer develop an appreciation of this pattern and the normal flow of speech and transfer the feeling to conversational speech.

Many therapists today in the field of speech and hearing have no prescribed therapeutic treatment for stuttering. Some say they just have the person slow down his speech, and this eliminates the problem. There are some who have the stutterer come into the office a few times a week for general conversation, etc. The stutterer begins to speak somewhat better in this situation, due to adaptation to the situation and to the therapist. It is hoped that he will then do as well outside the training facility.

Behavior modification and conditioning techniques have been used for years with every conceivable speech problem. The application of modern theory and therapy has taken on new connotations because of the vocabulary used in discussing its use. These procedures have been used in the treatment of stuttering in many different ways and are certainly not new.

A translation of the modern terms used in behavior modification to more familiar ones should bring a clearer understanding of the treatment suggested by behavior theorists.

Everyone is familiar with one or more techniques for promoting relaxation. Stimulus signals, and discriminative stimulus, all refer to preceding conditions or situations indicating the necessity for a response. With speech and the stutterer, these are conditions that require an oral response. Response is the speech that takes place as the result of the speaker's reaction to the cue to talk, with all of its related ramifications. Reinforcement is the positive or negative reward given to the speaker for whatever type of response he has made. In this case, desired responses or good speech is rewarded with praise or compliance with the speaker's request: positive reinforcement. Poor or undesirable responses result in a negative reaction or the withholding of a positive reward because of the stuttering. Positive reinforcement can be in the form of a pat on the back, or some other indication of approval as a reward.

Hiearchies are graded situations, usually from an event that produces little or no pressure or stress on the speaker, and progressing to those situations that make performance virtually an impossibility. This phenomenon is also noted to occur in stroke patients and others as it regards speech. Speech therapists were using desensitization long before modern behaviorists were in vogue. Progressive desensitization has been used to shape the speech behaviors of many different types of speaking problems as well as stuttering, progressively modifying the speech until the patient is able to perform in all types of speaking situations.

The preceding suggests that there has been wide usage of operant and classical conditioning in the treatment of stuttering. Behavior modification, as it is now used, reflects a highly organized and systematic approach to therapy. Much of what has been related above is utilized. Basically, the therapy is designed to progressively shape the desired behavior toward a prescribed goal. Behaviors leading to the goal are positively reinforced, while those that do not are negatively reinforced. A good behavior modification program calls for therapists and shapers of the behavior to work systematically and consistently toward the goal. This procedure is said to be effective in the remission of stuttering behavior, but some say that the process is too slow and of long duration.

Bloodstein (1949, 1950) reviewed the literature and listed those conditions under which the symptoms of stuttering were reduced:

1. Situations in which there is reduced communicative responsibility; for example, acting a role, speaking to an animal or child, talking with no-one present, or making an inconsequential remark.

2. Conditions in which there is minimal negative reaction to the stuttering by the listener, such as speaking to one's spouse or children, who are used to, and unconcerned about, the stuttering.

3. Experience of a change in the speech pattern. Changes in the rhythm pattern are extremely effective, especially singing, speaking in a singsong voice, speaking in time to a metronome, or reading in unison when the reading of the other acts as a pacemaker. Other changes in voice quality or intonation will also reduce the severity of stuttering quite markedly. Speaking as an accompaniment to rhythmic activity will also reduce the frequency of the stutterer.

4. Stuttering is reduced under conditions of unusual stimulation; in acute fear or anger, after the taking of some drugs, or during a loud noise when the stutterer cannot hear the sound of his own voice. Stuttering may be reduced by strong suggestion. Hypnotic suggestion may produce a striking temporary improvement in stuttering and even strong persuasion from some therapists may be effective.

The foregoing conditions and methods for reducing stuttering have been in use for many years by therapists and stuttering individuals themselves. There is a reduction in the stuttering, but there is no correction of the problem or transfer from one situation to others or permanence to the behavioral change.

Van Dantzig (1940) described speaking in regularly stressed syllables accompanied with tapping as a simple expedient for the relief of stuttering. She stated that in some this would be sufficient in itself, but in others it would have to be supplemented with other forms of therapy. This procedure is composed of two distractions, thought and motor.

The major emphasis in the treatment of stuttering today is directed toward having the stutterer learn as much as possible about how he stutters and what he does when stuttering occurs so that it can be modified (Boland, 1978). The major concern is with the repetitions, the hesitations, and the secondary symptoms in stuttering. Most therapies are directed toward alleviating the observable charactertistics of the problem and lessening some not so visible ones.

Much stress is given to improving the stutterer's attitude toward his problem and relieving his anticipations and anxieties. Some suggest that the fear of stuttering must be reduced or eliminated, so that the stutterer can learn to live with his problem and stutter more easily.

While many therapeutic procedures are advocated, none appear to suggest getting to the cause of the problem whatever it may be.

Many of the treatments advised are based on distracting the stutterer from the speech processes and speaking situations, thus affording him a crutch that will permit him to talk fluently for a period of time. The phenomenon of distraction was discussed earlier in this chapter.

Perhaps the most obvious aspect of the therapies suggested is that they all offer a substitution for normal speech. Except for a few treatment programs that offer a "cure for stuttering," the effect of therapy appears to be a continuation of stuttering but in a different way and in a way that is not as bad as the original problem.

For the stutterer, the implications have been that stuttering is with him always. There are some things that can be done to relieve some of the problems that appear, both physical and psychological, but according to current thinking, there is not too much that can be done about eliminating the problem; therefore, the stutterer must learn to live with his stuttering.

All but a few authorities reflect that they are not actually sure what causes stuttering, in the first place, and what perpetuates the problem after its original onset, in the second place.

Thus, without a definite cause and without agreement as to its perpetuation, there is no cure or correction for stuttering.

Summary

This chapter has dealt primarily with the therapeutic procedures that have been in vogue for many years and those of more recent origin. Treatments reviewed include distractions, psychoanalytic and psychological approaches, negative practice, voluntary stuttering, and others. More specific attention is given to the suggestions of Bloodstein, Boland, Eisenson, Glauber, Goldiamond, Johnson, Schwartz, Van Dantzig, Van Kirk, and Van Riper. The references noted résumés of their treatment theories. The publications of each would need to be read to obtain the full extent of their programs, beyond what is presented here.

Behavior modification and conditioning, as these procedures may apply to stuttering therapy, have been discussed in more historical terms with references made to the newer terminology. Hierarchies have been discussed as has been desensitization as it is applied to speech therapy.

The new concept in the treatment of stuttering, as suggested by *Self-Therapy for the Stutterer: One Approach* (1978) and apparently endorsed by many authorities in the field, also has been discussed.

Chapter 4

STUTTERING IS A SYNDROME

B Y DEFINITION from Dorland's *Medical Dictionary,* a syndrome is a set of symptoms that occur together, a symptom complex. Although syndromes are usually associated with a morbid state, referring to disease, stuttering has a possible neurological etiology and pathology, and its prognosis may be known or unknown. Stuttering is definitely a human problem with a complicated set of symptoms exhibited by those persons so involved. Many of the symptoms or behaviors are directly observable by the listener or diagnostician while others may go undetected by even the most experienced and professional observer. A point concerning semantics should be broached: a person is not a stutterer, he is a person with a problem of stuttering when he speaks.

Individuals exploring the problem of stuttering have tended to focus their attention on the observable symptoms. They have concentrated on the repetitious blocks and the behavioral variations perceived in persons who stutter and have approached the problem on the periphery and have not readily concerned themselves with underlying neurophysiological symptoms.

Stuttering is basically, from outward appearances, a speech problem in which the individual resorts to either repetitions of sound in words, or has prolongations, hesitations, or stoppages in initiating a particular speech sound. These variations can and do occur on the initial sound in words and on the first sound of a syllable anywhere in the word. Stuttering may occur with vowels and consonants.

STUTTERING BLOCKS

Stuttering blocks are clonic or tonic in nature. Clonic behaviors are those in which there is alternate contraction and relaxation of muscle groups in rapid succession. As an example, the person who stutters may make a series of *B*s: *B, B, B, B, B,* trying to initiate the initial sound in the word *bug.* The repetitive muscle patterns used to produce the sound *B* in this sequence of stuttering could be termed *clonic.*

Tonic behaviors are characterized by continuous tension. The prolongation of a vowel or consonant, as long *M——,* where the lip position and the phonation for *M* are continued for a period of time, longer than normal, in try to say a word as *May,* or holding the *ah* for *I* for an extended period of time, would be a tonic block. Tonic blocks also can take the form of continuous tensions, resulting in nothing being omitted. As on the sound *P* for *Pie,* the lips can be approximated, but the speaker cannot release the muscle contractions and let the air escape for the *P* sound.

Bilabial sounds are used as an example here. The problems, both clonic and tonic, can occur with any of the speech musculature. Such problems can involve the bilabial or lip muscles, muscles of the tongue, the mandible (jaw), the pharynx, and the larynx. Not only will the intrinsic musculature be implicated, but the extrinsic and associated muscles may be involved to one extent or another. As an illustration, the facial muscles are extrinsic to the lip muscles, and thus they would play a part in labial (lip) activity.

To continue the discussion concerning hesitations as tonic spasms or blocks, the laryngeal musculature may be involved in a tonic open position allowing the continued expulsion or exhalation of air, resulting in a lack of phonation for particular sounds. This same muscle group also could be implicated in a tonic spasm resulting in laryngeal closure with no air or sound being available for speech.

Stoppages, a term used by many to denote one of the observable behaviors in stuttering, would appear to be the result of a

tonic spasm or block.   In this instance, the muscle tensions would
result in the stopping of an articulated sound or the closing of
the vocal folds to occlude the flow of air for speech.

There is another source of trouble found in the person who
stutters: his breathing patterns have been noted to be deviant for
both quiet and speech breathing.

Examination of polygraph and kymograph recordings of normal speakers and those with stuttering problems reveals many
differences.   A majority of the persons who stutter have quiet
breathing patterns that are not synchronized when compared with
accepted norms.   Their patterns are usually marked with irregu-
larities in the time relationships of inhalation and exhalation.
There are quite often short inhalations followed by prolonged
exhalations.   The rhythm of the breathing is different in that
they may resort to a few rapid respiratory cycles; then, there will
be a period of apnea (no breathing) followed by a deep breath.
There is then a return to the pattern of short inspirations and
long expirations for a while, with the likelihood that the cycle
will begin again.   There are many variations that can be observed in the quiet breathing patterns of these people and noted
with considerable regularity.

In addition to the foregoing about quiet breathing, the abdominal-thoracic movements in the person who stutters are asynchronous.   There is a lack of phase relationship in the utilization
of this anatomy in respiration.   There are abdominal-thoracic reversals, with the chest going one way and the abdomen the other
during the in-and-out excursions associated with breathing.
There tends to be little consistency in the vasorhythms and the
breathing cycle as noted in normal speakers.   Normal breathing
will be explained in detail in the therapy section of this book.
Further analysis and comparisons of the two patterns will be
made in Chapter 6.

The person who stutters also has noticeable speech breathing
patterns.   Most of these individuals do inhale prior to speaking.
Some do not; they exhale, let all the air out, and then start to
speak.   The patterns of exhalation for speech show marked differences from those of normal speakers.   One obvious variation

is the presence of abdominal-thoracic reversals, mentioned above, which become more evident during speech. While he is speaking, the speech breathing patterns of the person who stutters are extensively blemished with such reversals, where the chest is depressed while the abodmen is protruded, creating a lack of phase relationship. This has a marked influence on speech. These breathing patterns are also marked with inspiratory gasps, when the individual will take in a quick breath out of phase, interrupting the exhalation of air for speech. Another deviation from normal speech breathing occurs during the initial release of air as speaking is initiated. Instead of waiting for the normal reciprocal movements of the breathing apparatus from inhalation to take place for speech, the person who stutters starts to speak before this occurs, thus depriving himself of this necessary transition. There are also those who take a breath, as mentioned above, let it all out, and try to talk on residual air that is not readily available for speech. Some are noted to have vital capacity (lung capacity) that is so limited that they are continually gasping and fighting for enough air to speak.

Although the variation in the breathing patterns of the person who stutters are quite obvious and are observable characteristics of the problem, rarely are they mentioned by those who write extensively about the cause, the signs, or the treatment of stuttering. Stuttering is not caused by irregular breathing patterns. These deviant patterns are symptoms of the problem and an outgrowth of underlying neurophysiological functions to be explained later.

HYPERTONUS

Another characteristic of stuttering is muscle tension or hypertonus. Most of the individuals who have the problem tend to be "tied-up in knots." The muscle tensions are not isolated to the speech muscles, but are apparent throughout the skeletal musculature including the legs, arms, trunk, and shoulder girdle, extending into those used for speech. Hypertonus is known to spread to all parts of the body when a person is tense for any reason. It is rare for a person to have muscle tension in only one isolated area or in one group of muscles without affecting the other muscles. The basic function of the nervous system would tend to preclude such isolation.

EMOTIONS

The person who stutters is involved emotionally with his speech problem. The emotional state is not the cause of the stuttering, but is the result of his own feelings and the reactions of others to his problem. Individuals who are emotionally disturbed due to anxiety and fear tend to have more hypertonus than those without such problems. Muscle tensions increase in the person who stutters whenever speech is anticipated or initiated. Although some muscle behaviors appear to be spasmodic cramping when secondary symptoms are observed, the level of tension does not actually develop to this extreme. However, there is an increase in tension during clonic and tonic stuttering blocks. Attempts to move the extremities of a stuttering individual reveal the degree of muscle tension he has throughout his body.

SECONDARY SYMPTOMS

Secondary symptoms are observed in almost all adolescent and adult persons who stutter and are occasionally seen in younger children, depending on how involved their stuttering problem has become. Secondary symptoms have been described and defined as many different things from ticlike behaviors to any unnatural movements or mannerisms made or exhibited while a person is stuttering, without reference to any abnormal activity in the speech mechanism. However, such symptoms do appear in the speech mechanism in various forms.

Secondary symptoms are superfluous observable and unobservable behaviors that are an outgrowth of what the person who stutters resorts to in a vain attempt to relieve his stuttering. Many of these symptoms are muscle or motor behaviors that can be seen by the observer. They tend to range from simple eye blinking to turning the eyes away. Symptoms may include facial grimacing or contortions, averting the head, or protruding the tongue. There can be minimal to excessive movements of the hand and arms that include wiggling, tapping, or snapping the fingers; waving, extending, flexing, and describing various figures, and assuming distorted postures with the arms. Excessive leg and foot movements may be noted, such as shuffling the feet, tapping a foot, extending or flexing the legs, or assuming bizarre leg postures. These behaviors can develop to the extent that the individual will resort to extreme body contortions that include the face, head, tongue, shoulders, arms, trunk, and legs in an attempt to break out of or through a stuttering block. There are times when the symptoms appear to be painful. In spite of all this, the individual still stutters.

Unobservable secondary symptoms usually can be detected by the experienced speech pathologist, but there are therapists who fail to note these problems. Such symptoms include alterations in the breathing patterns that may take on various forms. A person may resort to an unnatural release of air to start his speech. (This is recommended by some as a correction for stuttering.) There may be, and often are, inspiratory gasps of air that punctuate the exhalation phase of breathing for speech. Some will attempt to speak during inspiration or inhalation of air. Several breaths may be taken, and then an attempt will be made to initiate speech. There are many variations of these symptoms. Since no two persons tend to have identical problems when it comes to stuttering, it would appear appropriate for there to be many and wide variations in the distractions used and the secondary symptoms acquired.

Another unobserved symptom is the use of synonyms to replace words with which the person who stutters anticipates difficulty. This may also be the device used to avoid a particular speech phoneme on which the person is sure that he will stutter. In order to evade certain words or sounds with which he has difficulty, the individual will anticipate their usage and quickly sidestep them by selecting another word having the same or nearly the same meaning. This is common practice in adults and some adolescents.

Secondary symptoms are the behaviors being used and the

residual of those that have been used as distractions to keep from stuttering. Unfortunately, there does not seem to be any attempt to abandon a worn-out distraction that has become a secondary symptom when a new distraction is adopted. To the contrary, the pattern seems to be to add the newest distraction to those that have been used before, even though the old ones have lost their effectivness as distracting agents. This results in a procedure whereby the stuttering problem keeps getting bigger, more complicated, and worse because of the accumulation of distractions and secondary symptoms. Secondary problems begin when the involved individual becomes aware of his stuttering and tries to do something about it.

Therapy or treatment techniques can easily be adopted by the stuttering person as distractions and eventually become secondary symptoms. This tends to occur if the person feels that a certain procedure will help his speech. He then focuses his attention on it rather than resorting to normal speech behaviors. Nothing more is needed to start the process than a suggestion from the therapist or practitioner that a particular technique or procedure will help or cure his stuttering. The naive therapist, psychologist, or any other person working with individuals with stuttering problems often makes such suggestions. There may be temporary relief from stuttering for a period of time, but usually, when the distraction begins to lose its effectiveness, it will not be abandoned; it will be maintained as a part of the symptom complex.

Secondary symptoms do not cause stuttering, nor are they stuttering. They are secondary characteristics of the problem brought on either by the individual in his attempts to help himself or by what others have told him to do to eliminate his stuttering and improve his speaking ability.

STUTTERING VERSUS CLUTTERING

There have been some who have stated that stuttering resembles cluttering in that the person who stutters tends to speak rapidly. It is the opinion of this author that the rapid rates of speech, used by individuals who stutter or clutter, are two different phenomena. Throughout the many years of experience and five years as the director and the head speech pathologist of the Neurological Diagnostic Unit of the Institute of Logopedics (1967-1972), he saw or examined only a few individuals who could actually be said to clutter.

Cluttering, to this author, is speaking at such a rapid rate that the speech becomes unintelligible. In this discourse there are some definite patterns that are observed. Besides the very rapid rate of speaking, there are distortions and omissions of speech phonemes. Syllables are omitted in multisyllable words. Words are omitted as the person rushes headlong through phrases and sentences. Breathing patterns are usually short with a low vital capacity for speech.

The basis for cluttering is undoubtedly neurophysiological and may be related to a lack of control of thought to speech output. As will be noted later in Chapter 5, thought-to-speech output occurs very rapidly. If the thought patterns are extremely rapid and the individual is trying to think out loud, or speak as fast as he is thinking, these processes could readily account for the rapidity in motor behavior. The speech musculature cannot function as rapidly as the individual's thoughts, and only bits and pieces of the desired speech output are possible. This is speculation on the part of the author at this time.

The rapid rate of speech noted in the person who stutters is an entirely different phenomenon, and for separate reasons. There is a wide range of variability in the rate of speaking of those who stutter. At times the rate may be slow and rather deliberate; at other times the rate of speech may be normal. The rapid speech rate is found to occur between stuttering blocks. Usually there will be a block of some type, then a rapid flow of speech until the next block occurs or he stops speaking.

It is noted and reported by those who stutter that at times the way looks clear, nothing is coming up to give them any concern. Their desire is to get it said before something that might give them trouble, a word or a sound, does appear on the horizon. In these instances, they rush ahead with what they want to say. The speech then comes out in spurts or spasmodic utterances.

It will be noted that these utterances or periods of speaking rapidly are coherent. The words and sentences are complete. The articulation of speech is normal, provided that the person does not have any articulatory disorder along with the stuttering problem. Most often there is no lack of breath for speaking. He just sees a clear road ahead and "takes off." In most instances he is rushing headlong into the next tonic or clonic stuttering block.

Summary

Stuttering is a human speech problem with a complicated set of symptoms. It is a syndrome because of the set of diagnostic symptoms or symptom complex exhibited by those persons involved. The symptoms have been identified and discussed. The nature of stuttering has been discussed relative to the types of muscle spasms noted. Reference has been made to the nature of the muscle behaviors found in stuttering and termed *clonic* and *tonic* spasms or blocks. Laryngeal valving and breathing problems are found to be defective. Hypertonus is a total body phenomenon and not an isolated muscle problem. Distractions tend to become secondary symptoms; they embellish and further complicate the stuttering problem. Any therapy technique or procedure can become a distraction.

Stuttering is not caused by breathing problems or by emotional disturbances. Secondary symptoms are not stuttering, nor do they cause stuttering; they just make the problem worse. Stuttering and cluttering are different problems.

Chapter 5

A NEW LOOK AT THE OLD PROBLEM

IT APPEARS THAT, throughout the course of history, mankind has been concerned with the cause and effect of everything. He has forever been exploring what gives rise to the forces of nature, the origin of disease and illness, what occasions aging and other mysteries of life. Man also has been exploring the cause of stuttering, possibly since the problem was first noticed. Many theories, philosophies, and speculations have been proffered with no one arriving at a true etiology as yet. Perhaps one will never be found.

Causes for stuttering have ranged from possible damage to the nervous system to possible psychological and psychiatric etiologies, to "just naming it causes it." Most modern theories seem to be speculations by psychologists and psychiatrists. Most speech pathologists who have offered their thinking also have had strong psychological backgrounds. Members of the medical community are apparently too busy keeping human beings in good health to wonder and hypothesize about a possible cause of stuttering.

Most of the theories advanced have been based on observations of the symptoms of the problem. From these observations, hypotheses have been put together, mostly based on assumptions that this must be the way it is from the way it looks and how the person acts and reacts in speaking situations. In groups from which a consensus of opinion has been derived, it appears that the first order of business has been to agree to agree.

There have been isolated instances where an individual has proclaimed that he has solved the problem. The solutions appear to have been attempts to solve the riddle of one of the symptoms of stuttering, as so often happens. In solving these riddles, much incorrect information has been formulated. In most instances, the solution for the elimination of the symptom did not solve the problem because then another symptom had to be solved, one unrelated to the first symptom. None of the solutions for resolving the symptoms has resulted in an understanding as to the cause of stuttering or to its complete remediation.

This author has based his thinking on the fact that the person who stutters is not ill. He is not the victim of an insult to his nervous system. Psychologically, the period from two to four years of age is not a time when ego-id conflicts predominate. The child has not developed a neurosis or psychosis. He is not overly concerned by the labels placed on things and tends to accept things at face value, although he is developing some inquisitiveness concerning cause and effect. He is into the "why age."

It is firmly believed that the child who has nonfluencies between the ages of two and four years is a perfectly normal, healthy child. The largest percentage of children passing through this age do have nonfluencies. It is hardly reasonable to assume that better than 50 percent of all children passing through this stage of development and displaying some repetitions, etc., in their speech have one of the problems mentioned above. Only 1 percent of the population continues to have the problem beyond the age of five years. There has to be another answer.

Children progressing through the ages from two to four years have many problems if comparisons are made with those who are one to two years older. A close examination of their motor behaviors reveals numerous "problems," whereas, in reality, the behaviors are perfectly normal for this age range.

An evaluation of the average two to four year old child's ambulatory and other leg behaviors shows that he is a clumsy person. He can walk, go up and down stairs, and run fairly well. These are all very gross motor behaviors. He cannot kick, skip, hop, nor can he dance with any degree of specific muscle control. (The muscle behaviors used in these activities do not require the same level of synergic controls required for more refined movements.) More central nervous system development must occur before these actions are possible. The muscle controls and levels of development are normal for this age, but behind those of slightly older children.

Next, take a sample of the child's hand or manual behaviors. The two to four year old can perform some motor acts requiring fairly good control. He can feed himself and partially dress himself. Finger control is not advanced far enough to tie shoes or handle small buttons, hooks and eyes. He has difficulty drawing the simplest geometric figures, a circle or a square, if at all. Controls are decidedly lacking in the use of crayon or pencil. He does not have sufficient control of the hand and arm to stay within the lines of the picture being colored. One-handed tasks present some problems, but two-handed activities are even less developed and reflect gross inadequacies. He may be able to catch a ball, but it is done very clumsily and most often missed. The slightly older child, ages five and six, is doing better because his nervous system has developed just that much more. The muscles used in controlling movements of the hand, fingers, and arms are not so large as those in the legs and require more nervous system control to perform the many refined motor skills that will have to be learned as the child grows older.

The two to four year old is learning to talk. His vocabulary is gradually expanding from approximately 275 words at the age of two to 1550 words by the time he is four years old. He is acquiring the speech phonemes of his language, slowly but surely, and will not have them all mastered until he is at least five years old.

The child is beginning to put words together to make phrases and sentences. At the age of two years, his mean number of words per response is 1.8. By the age of four years, his mean number of words per response is 4.4 words. The child will use longer responses, but the average length of his phrases and sentences will be as given here. At two years of age much of his speech will be unintelligible: he mispronounces many words, particularly multisyllables that require more muscle synthesis and fine motor control. Time and further nervous system control will improve these behaviors.

The child has been using the muscles for sucking, chewing, and swallowing to ingest nourishment from two to four years. He is not quite able to handle all foods with a refined level of dexterity. He still has some problems with his tongue, lips, pharynx, and muscles of the jaw. His meat must be cut into small pieces. He consumes soft foods with greater dispatch than hard, chewy foods. Even these behaviors are in the period of development. It will be a while before he is a skillful eater.

In learning to speak, the child will need to use the same muscles that he has used for eating, with the addition of those for respiration and phonation. There are not different sets of muscles for eating and speaking (producing the articulated movements for speech sounds); they are the same. The muscles used in eating and speaking are much smaller and require much more refined control to perform their specific activities than do the larger muscles of the body. The muscle movements for speech must be very precise, and the timing must be exact. Slight variations in the synchronization of all of the muscles used in speech can distort the patterns in many ways. There can be defectively articulated phonemes. There may be substitutions, omissions, deviations, and additions of the sounds used in speaking. Such defects fall into a wide variety of problems.

The production of phonation for certain speech phonemes necessitates the coordination of the breathing musculature and the muscles of the larynx. Add to this the phenomena where the sound or phonation must be turned on and off as required for phonation or just an airstream for the production of different speech sounds. This operation has to be synchronized with the movements of the tongue, lips, jaw, the soft palate, etc. Speech, it appears, demands the acme of human muscle systematization for its proper output. These muscle behaviors with this requisite of synergy for speaking do not just happen; they are initiated, guided, and controlled by the nervous system.

In the two to four year old child and even in older children, seven years and older, the nervous system is still in the process of development. The cerebral cortex and lower neural centers have further growth and maturation to experience before the system is fully developed and able to control the muscle behaviors necessary for the development of advanced human skills. Refined motor skills, as they are known, do not develop until the child is seven years old or older and continue to develop into adult life.

The portion of the nervous system involved in controlling the motor activities of the human being is the cerebellum. The synergic controls necessary for such behaviors are organized in this area of neurophysiology. According to Grinker and Bucy (1949), ". . . the cerebellum is the organ by which the cerebral cortex achieves integrative synergia in voluntary movement."

A better understanding of synergy and the functions of the cerebellum can best be appreciated by observing the results of damage to it. The concern will center on asynergia. The neo-cerebellum is the site of the classic asynergic syndrome.

Elliott (1969) has written the following:

> Asynergia (Gk. non-together-acting) is the true motor defect and involves a more severe degree of cerebellar loss. It means that the subject cannot perform movements smoothly and efficiently even when he is watching them. He can, indeed, carry out any desired movement — he is not paralysed in any proper sense of the word; but he must control each muscle by conscious effort. When one considers the many elements that must be swiftly and precisely coordinated in even the most routine acts, such as walking, the gravity of this condition is understandable. All motor response is clumsy, faltering, jerky and tremulous; the subject is easily exhausted by the extra effort and attention required to achieve even crude coordination; . . . Injury to the cerebellar cortex obliterates the motor patterns recorded there and abolishes the means for "computing" new patterns. . . . Injury to the more compact internal nuclei, through which practically all outflow is channeled, has characteristically more severe effects; and injury to the efferent tracts has the most severe effects of all — even if the cortex with its control patterns is intact, its influence cannot play on the motor pool.

Some of the subsymptoms that are of interest are past pointing, rebound, and the inability to carry out repeated rhythmic movements. All of the symptoms of the asynergic syndrome can be derived from the basic defect in muscle coordination.

Another reference of interest concerning the cerebellum, this time the paleocerebellum, has pointed out that there are visceral connections, sympathetic and parasympathetic. The effects are produced through or by way of hypothalamic connections. These connections may be of importance when investigating the effects emotions may play on motor activities, breathing, etc. In spite of the vast amount of research that has been done on the cerebellum, "half of the cerebellum or more is uncommitted. All of this area is neocerebellar and purely cerebral afferents which come from the cortical areas (frontal and parietal association cortex) without known functional topology" (Elliott, 1969).

For years the cerebellum was thought of as being involved in such problems as decerebrate rigidity, maintaining orientation under vestibular guidance, the integration of proprioception of the limbs, and the unsymmetrical movements conducted by the cerebral cortex. More recently, the function of the cerebellar cortex has been found to be extremely important in all motor activities.

Elliott (1969) stated the findings of Ruch (1965) and Snider and Stowell (1944). The cerebellum is neither sensory nor motor, but is a correlation center. It gives rise neither to sensation nor to overt movement. It correlates the muscle, tendon-vestibular messages reaching it and tactile, visual, and auditory elements. On the basis of the information received, "it computes the most effective deployment of muscular effort to perform a required movement. It then brings the resultant to bear on the motor neuron pool and on the motor cortex itself. It sensitizes or facilitates in such a way that a cerebral discharge to the pool will set off a well-integrated response."

Ruch (1965) suggested that "the cerebellar cortex forms one end of a cerebro-cerebellar circuit; in this, it has the function of programming cerebral motor control in time-sequence." It acts as a storehouse of patterns and fires a sequence of instructions to the cerebrum. "It would thus regulate the timing and composition of an action."

The cerebellum has been divided into three regions according to evolutionary stages. These divisions are (1) the archicerebellum, (2) the paleocerebellum, and (3) the neocerebellum. It is necessary to consider only the neocerebellum for the purposes being manifested in this writing.

Elliott (1969) has made this statement:

> The neocerebellum is evidently a highly educable organ. The patterns for special skills are certainly not present at birth must be slowly incorporated by the child-or an adult learning a new technic. . . . The patterns once incorporated, discharge in such a way as to guide the cerebrum along established channels of action — though the cerebrum adapts the action to circumstances; and at the same time they "set" the motor pool so as to facilitate the action.

It is not intended, in this manuscript, to burden the reader with an enormous amount of neurology and neurophysiology. The neural connections between the cerebellum and the cerebral cortex will be given to familiarize the reader or student with this most important part of the central nervous system and to assist in conducting him through the reasoning of this author in arriving at the postulate being presented.

The most modern afferent paths or tracts to the cerebellum are the cortico-ponto-cerebellar tracts. Great numbers of fibers come from extensive areas of the cerebral cortex. They form two separate tracts, one from the prefrontal and premotor cortex, the fronto-pontine. The other tract is from the parietal lobe, the parieto-pontine. The complete names of these tracts would be the parieto-occipito-temporo-pontine. "These tracts run in the cerebral peduncles to end in the pons. Secondary fibers run through the brachium pontis to the cerebellar cortex" (Elliott, 1969).

From the cerebellar cortex, axons of Purkinje cells run to the internal nuclei of the same organ. Then, secondary fibers course through the brachium conjunctivum, through the midbrain to the nucleus ventralis of the thalamus. From here, fibers run to the precentral cortex, areas 4 and 6. These are the cerebello-cerebral connections (Elliott, 1969).

In simpler terms, there are tracts or nerves coming from the various areas of the cerebral cortex not involved in the projection of motor outflow. These tracts come from association or silent areas of the brain and are involved in receiving messages from inside and outside the body. These regions are comprised of the frontal, parietal, temporal, and occipital lobes of the cerebral hemispheres. Areas of these lobes are concerned with receiving information through the senses, and deciphering and interpreting the information received. They are the areas in which thinking takes place, making decisions, and determining the actions that should or should not be made in response to sensory stimuli.

For speech, these are areas involved in receiving and understanding. Their function is also to construct the responses or messages to be sent or spoken, the questions and the answers. If the decision is to respond with a motor response, which speech definitely is, the message is sent to the cerebellum by way of the tract mentioned above, the cerebro-cerebellar pathways.

The cerebellum is like a large computer that receives the information to act in a motor way. It computes the motor behaviors from muscle movements or patterns that have been learned, and sends the resultant or computer readout to the motor cortex. The motor cortex is a project area of the brain from which nerve impulses are "fired," so to speak, to initiate muscle actions. The cerebral motor cortex carries out the motor behavior as specified by the cerebellum.

The cerebellum is a storehouse of learned or acquired muscle patterns, actions, behaviors, etc., that have been learned or programmed in its cells. Voluntary motor responses are ordered by the cerebral cortex. They are computed, programmed, and initiated by the cerebellum. The finalized or computed information concerning the nature of the motor action is forwarded to the motor cortex, which follows the program.

No neurophysiological activity is quite this simple because there is extensive interaction of all facets of the central and peripheral nervous systems in most human behaviors. The interplay between the cerebellum and the cerebral cortex described above will be sufficient for this undertaking.

Taking what has just been stated above as the basis for voluntary motor responses or actions, an application to and for speech is the next step in the reasoning process followed in the new look at stuttering.

Speech is the most complicated, difficult, integrated voluntary muscle behavior performed by human beings. Most of the muscles employed in speaking are small, with the largest muscles being used for respiration. Speaking utilizes the muscles of the lips, jaw, tongue, soft palate or velum, pharynx, larynx, and those of the thorax, diaphragm, and abdomen. Add to these the extrinsic muscles that assist in the activities of the organs previously mentioned, and a person will be using muscles of the trunk, neck and face, etc., for speech. This would tend to exclude only the musculature of the arms and legs from the speaking process. The actions of the muscles and muscle groups involved must be highly synchronized for speech to be appropriately emitted.

Keeping the foregoing information in mind concerning the functions of the cerebral cortex and cerebellum, one finds that speech appears to be accomplished in the following manner. The association areas of the cortex are involved in receiving sensory stimuli, words, etc., deciphering them, and abstracting their meanings. These areas are concerned with the thinking processes that occur. The person decides what he wishes to say. This message is sent to the cerebellum, which programs the muscle behaviors necessary to send the message to speak. The muscle activities for the articulation of speech phonemes (as they have been learned and stored) and the associated motor behaviors of breathing and laryngeal valving (phonation) are computed. The resultant or planned program is neurophysiologically transmitted to the cerebral motor cortex. The giant Betz cells are excited or stimulated and initiate the muscle actions as planned.

The human appears to be programmed for speech as he has learned it. If he has a defective speech phoneme, he learned it that way and it will be so programmed until he is reprogrammed, or learns to do it correctly. (There will be more about speech later.)

In order not to leave the impression that the processes involved in any motor activity are as simple as outlined above, it must be stated that the impulse patterns discharged through any final efferent (motor) axon are determined by the summation of a myriad of different forces, the highest expression of the central nervous system. In the final analysis, the state of each unit is the result of countless conditions, past and present, in the periphery of the organism, in the lower neural centers, in the thalamus, and in all the rest of the cortex (Elliott, 1969).

In continuing to establish the basis for the new look at stuttering, it is necessary to evaluate the function and growth of the cerebellum as far as medical research has provided the information.

It will be recalled that earlier in this chapter reference was made to the three developmental-functional divisions of the cerebellum. It is essential that they be considered briefly as regards their growth.

According to Elliott (1969), "The Archicerebellum is primitive in all respects. . . . In the human fetus it differentiates first and its white matter myelinates first." It is concerned largely with vestibular matters.

The paleocerebellum myelinates, and so becomes functional, late in the human infant — which may correlate with the late development of voluntary control over the limbs.

The neocerebellum develops late in the fetus, but its myelination apparently begins fairly soon after birth. It becomes overwhelmingly dominant in man, supremely so. It is mainly under cerebral control, but also olivary control. It is "the region that receives connections only from these organs."

The foregoing would appear to suggest that the neocerebellum of the two to four year old has developed to some degree but its myelinization is not complete, and thus its function is limited. It also would seem that the programming of the neocerebellum has barely begun. It is in an early stage of neurological development. The child is learning motor behaviors that will be stored, but altered and improved upon as his nervous system grows and develops, and becomes more extensively myelinated.

Speaking is a motor behavior. The child is just learning how to talk. There are many speech sounds for which he has not learned the motor behaviors by the age of two years. He will learn the motor behaviors for these sounds during the next two to three years.

The two year old is incorporating more and more words into his vocabulary. His vocabulary of understanding far exceeds his vocabulary of expression, but it will grow rapidly from about 200 words at age two to approximately 5,000 by ages five to six.

The two year old is starting to put words together, to make phrases and sentences that are functionally complete but structurally incomplete. The average length of his responses is two words. As he grows toward four and five years of age, his phrases and sentences will become more structurally complete, and his average length of response will be four words or more.

Thus, for the two to four year old child, this period of development is permeated with the acquisition of the refined and highly synchronized motor activities required for speech.

The new look at the initial onset of stuttering is that the problem is a manifestation of the developmental level of the nervous system, namely the cerebellum, between the ages of two and four years. The cerebellum is not yet able to handle adequately or satisfactorily the flow of messages from the association areas of the cerebral cortex and convert them into refined, synergic muscle patterns to be carried out by the cerebral motor cortex.

Fay (1953) stated that the synergic control of speech patterns was in the cerebellum. Thus, with a primitive, undeveloped, inadequately programmed cerebellum, the repetitions and/or prolongations, the clonic and tonic muscle patterns noted in a young child's speech are a natural phenomenon.

It appears that cerebellar development is such that the period of normal tonic and clonic muscle behaviors in speech is short-lived. Development, storing, and programming appear to go hand in hand so that the child seemingly outgrows his problem in a span of two to three years. There is no damage here, no neurosis; actually, no problem. This is a normal stage in the child's development of speech.

It must be noted that during this same developmental period other motor behaviors also greatly improve. Hopping, skipping, using scissors, drawing geometric figures, and staying within the lines while coloring have all improved. There are still improvements to be made before these muscle behaviors are well learned and become refined motor skills, but the child is progressing as he should.

But what about stuttering that continues after the age of four or five years? Most children have had a period of nonfluency and have realized the effects of further development of the cerebellum and no longer have the problem. Approximately 1 to 2 percent of the two to four year old population does not gain normal fluent speech. The question is, What happens? Why does a particular child continue to stutter or have nonfluencies? Why does the problem exist with some individuals for a lifetime?

According to information gathered from persons who stutter at every level, child, adolescent, and adult, the delineation is the same. Somewhere, somehow, and sometimes under unknown conditions, stuttering developed. These individuals stopped behaving as normal speakers in regard to their thought-to-speech behavior. What turned them around could have been many things. A look, a sharp reprimand, an expressed or unexpressed concern, mimicry on the part of others, a sudden self-realization, or "what have you" could have been the turning point.

The turning point, as perceived by this author, is when the child ceases to think and talk as a normal speaker. In normal speakers, the thought-to-speech output is such that there is no perceptible delay between thinking what is to be said and saying it. The transition from the "thought to be spoken" to the resultant of the computed program of that thought into motor speech output appears to be instantaneous. There is a very short delay between thought and speaking, but the nervous impulse travels so fast — approximately 120 meters per second — that the time interval is not discernible. The impression is that, when one is speaking, thoughts become speech instantly, like "thinking-out-loud." No thought has to be given to articulatory movements, breathing, laryngeal valving, etc.; it all happens for you. The motor aspects of speaking are computed and programmed through the cerebellum to the cerebral motor cortex.

The person who continues to stutter is the child who has a thought-to-speech behavior change. This change can occur at any age and at any time, but the two to four year old is more susceptible because of the nonfluencies he is having at the time. The change in thought-to-speech behavior begins when the child starts to think ahead, thinking of what he wants to say during the time he is already talking. While he is speaking, the individual is planning what he wants to say next. What he is saying at a given moment is what he thought of previously while he was saying something else.

All people think when they talk, but they do not think words ahead, nor do they think sentences or even paragraphs ahead while trying to speak at the same time. This is what the person who stutters tends to do.

The child may think only a few words ahead while the older child and the adolescent may do the same with a sentence. The adult may think anywhere from a sentence to a paragraph ahead. These individuals do not have consistent, concurrent thought-to-speech patterns. Their thoughts and speech are not occurring at the same time. Speaking is behind or delayed in relation to thinking; or, to turn it around, thinking is far ahead of talking. The person who continues to stutter has thinking and speech output that is out of phase. Because these two behaviors are out of phase, confusion prevails.

As was noted earlier, there are direct neural connections between the association or silent areas of the cerebral cortex, the parietal lobe, etc., and the cerebellum. It is the opinion of this author that there is a confusing state of affairs concerning messages to the cerebellum in terms of what is desired in the way of motor behaviors for speech output. The cerebellum, as a computer, becomes jammed, so to speak, so that phase relations are disturbed and muscle behaviors for speech are lacking in synergy. As a result of these conditions, there are repetitions, hesi-

tations, prolongations, and stoppages in the muscle patterns programmed for speech. It is believed that this is the prime reason
for the continuation of stuttering after the problem should have
been overcome as the cerebellum continued to develop.

In reciting rote materials such as the days of the week, numbers, months of the year, nursery rhymes, etc., individuals state
that they do not have to think ahead. The speech just comes
out. The same seems to apply to frequently used phrases, emotionally toned responses, and to profanity. Most persons who
stutter do not have problems with this type of material. Singing adds new elements to the vocal utterances such as a melody,
a marked rhythm, and different variations in accent. While
singing, the singer must maintain a normal thought-to-song output if all of the components of the lyrics and music, etc., are to
be executed correctly. Talking to oneself is another behavior
that is done without thinking ahead. These changes in thought-
to-speech behavior have been reported by children, adolescents,
and adults who stutter. They also report that, if they first think
of what they want to say when not speaking, and then say it, it
comes out fluently because they are not thinking ahead during
speech output.

It is well documented that changes in the propositional levels
affect the speaking performance of the person who stutters. The
higher the value the individual places on the occasion, or circumstances, the more he will stutter. The greater the pressure in
the situation in which he must speak, the more he thinks ahead
in an attempt to select the most acceptable or appropriate things
to say. The lower the level or propositionality or pressure he
feels the less thought he gives to what he wants to say. As he
grows older, he uses "thinking ahead" to intercept sounds and
words with which he foresees difficulty, and then resorts to using
other words if possible. This type of anticipation, related to
thinking ahead, becomes a secondary symptom, mostly in the
adolescent and the adult who stutter.

Secondary symptoms are all of the extra motor and thought
behaviors to which the person who stutters resorts, in a vain
attempt to relieve his stuttering. By engaging in these actions he

distracts himself to the extent that he stops thinking ahead. The problem is that the distraction does not work very long, it loses its distracting effect, and then usually becomes just another secondary symptom that makes the enigma greater. Thus, the problem of stuttering becomes compounded as the person tries to do something about his difficulty. At this stage, he has a chronic, habitual stuttering problem.

The foregoing information has dealt primarily with the most observable aspects of stuttering: the repetitions, hesitations, and prolongations that occur while speaking. Consideration should now be given to those behaviors that are involved in the speech process, but are not readily discernible: breathing and laryngeal valving.

In Chapter 4 it was noted that the person with a stuttering problem had deviant quiet and speech breathing patterns. They were listed as symptoms of the stuttering syndrome. To review the behaviors, these individuals had quiet breathing patterns that were asynchronous and out of phase with the cardiac rhythms; the inhalation-exhalation or inspiratory-expiratory aspects of quiet respiration were faulty in that the inhalation phase of the cycle was shorter than that for exhalation; and the phases were not symmetrical. In some instances there tended to be abdominal-thoracic reversals during quiet breathing.

The person who stutters also was found to have deviant speech breathing patterns. He did not wait or allow for the normal change or reversal of the respiratory muscle patterns from inhalation to exhalation of air for speaking. The exhalation phase of breathing for speech was marked with inspiratory gasps and abdominal-thoracic reversals during which the thorax is depressed while the abdomen is distended.

Respiration is a survival mechanism controlled by the sympathetic and parasympathetic nervous systems and is influenced by the oxygen–carbon dioxide ratio in the blood. The actual process of breathing is the result of the functions of the muscles of respiration. It appears that, during the act of speaking, the breathing activities may be taken over, so to speak, by the cerebellum as a speech-related activity. This would account for the synergy that must occur between the muscles of respiration and the muscles of the tongue, lips, and jaw responsible for the articulatory movements in normal speech. It appears that laryngeal valving, speech breathing, and the muscle behaviors for the articulation of speech are all coordinated in the same manner. It would seem plausible that the problems associated with cortical-cerebellar interactions, as previously noted, also would affect these major aspects of speech output in the person who stutters.

If all of the musculature involved in speech production is computed, programmed, and the resultant relayed by way of the cerebellum to the cerebral motor cortex, as suggested in this writing, and if the synergic controls for speaking are out of phase to the extent that they involve all of the muscle patterns that must be synchronized for normal fluency, then the early nonfluencies of children must be the result of a normal developmental phenomenon. The continuation of nonfluencies beyond the normal age for their remission may be the result of what has happened to the person and his thought-to-speech behaviors and their effect on the flow of muscle activities that produce the spoken word.

A question arises concerning the cycling phenomenon that appears to occur in stuttering. There are periods of time when the child who stutters will have what is apparently normal, fluent speech. These periods of fluency do not seem to appear so readily for the older adolescent or the adult person who stutters. There is no consistency to the periods or cycles of fluent speech. They seem to occur at random and are of varying duration. It appears that during the fluent cycles the child who stutters has his thought-to-speech behavior straightened out and is performing as a normal speaker. For some reason he has righted the wrong that has prevailed. He will continue to be a fluent speaker until something happens to draw his attention again to his speech; at this time he will revert to his stuttering and his thinking-ahead behavior.

He is now paying too much attention to his speech and is in trouble, at least for a while. If he could maintain a reasonably long period of fluent speech and normal thought-to-speech behavior, he probably would not return to stuttering. This, how-ever, is very unlikely because of the reactions of his peers, his family, and others in his environment who would and usually do react unfavorably toward his return to nonfluent speech. His greatest problem is with himself. Normal speakers occasionally will trip over a word and have a hesitation, or a repetition, but they think nothing of it and go on talking in their usual way. This is not so with the person who has stuttered. If he has even the slightest problem, he will revert to previous habits that bring on his stuttering.

The person who does not continue to stutter did not become the victim of the thought-to-speech change. He had his period of nonfluency and, as his cerebellum developed and became more capable of handling thought-to-speech assignments, his fluent speech returned.

Summary

The proposed new look at the old problem of stuttering has been presented. The cerebellum has been suggested as the area of the central nervous system most probably involved in the ini-tial phase of nonfluent speech because of its level of development and insufficient programming capabilities to handle the onslaught of speech behavior demanded by the human through his cerebral cortex. The continuation of nonfluencies has been related to a change in thought-to-speech behavior that appears to affect the function of the cerebellum in its attempts to program the muscle behaviors for speech output. The various symptoms of stutter-ing have been accounted for in this premise. It is felt by this author that most, if not all, of the questions that have surfaced concerning stuttering have been answered here. Whether they actually have been answered adequately may be determined only by further investigation of the nervous system, utilization of the hypothesis presented here, and time.

Chapter 6

THE ESTABLISHMENT OF MORE NORMAL
SPEECH BEHAVIOR

THE NEW LOOK at the old problem of stuttering has been reviewed with its application to all of the symptoms and characteristics of the problem. There remains now the necessity to design a rehabilitation program that will reduce or eliminate the
symptoms and characteristics of stuttering and help to advance
normal speaking behavior. First, consideration must be given to
a workable definition of what constitutes normal speech. What
is normal thought-to-speech behavior, and what neurophysiological processes are involved?

Normal speech is apparently difficult to define. A review of
some literature revealed that definitions ranged from a simple
"speech is the utterance of vocal sounds conveying ideas" (Dorland's, 1962) to a rather long definition from West and Ansberry
(1968) in which they elaborate on four aspects of speech: linguis-
tic, phonatory, articulatory, and auditory. They do say that
speech is "formalized oral communication." Many authors offer
definitions of deviant or defective speech in preference to defin-
ing normal speech.

For current considerations, it may be said that normal speech
is the process of conveying an idea from one human being to
another by way of orally articulated symbols or sounds in a time
scheme and in such manner that the ideas are exchanged and received as intended. The general nature of the manner of normal, articulated speech is determined by the locale of the speaker
and whether or not the speech sounds fall within the accepted
norms for the geographical area. Normal speech is usually con-

sidered to be void of substitutions, omissions, distortions, or additions of speech phonemes. It is also judged to be smooth flowing without repetitions, hesitations, prolongations, etc. There are other aspects that could be included, but they are not of concern in this writing.

In the new look at stuttering, the process of thought-to-speech was given considerable review in that it was reasoned that persons who continued to stutter, after the time of normal remission of stuttering, did not conform to normal thinking-to-speaking behaviors. The normal process of thinking-to-speaking is almost like thinking "out loud." The person speaking is thinking, but the interval between the thought and the output of that thought as speech is so rapid that the speaker is unable to detect the delay time.

It must be recalled that nerve impulses travel at extremely high rates of speed. The transmission of a thought from the cerebral cortex to the cerebellum and back to the cerebral motor cortex required only a fraction of a second. The flow of thoughts that are to be spoken is usually rapid also. Thus, with the rapidity of thought combined with the speed of those thoughts to speech output, the individual, for all practical purposes, is "thinking out loud."

In speaking, the individual does not have to concern himself with the many facets of speech output. He does not have to stop and think about the muscle patterns needed to produce the articulatory movements. It is not necessary for him to consciously control the opening and closing of the larynx as phonated and nonphonated speech phonemes are formed. He need not worry about his breathing patterns, etc. These behaviors are all stored, programmed, and computed, as needed for output, by the cerebellum. All that the individual has to do is to decide to talk, start the process of thought-to-speech, and speech is emitted. The muscle behavior patterns are "automatic," so to speak. Thought patterns initiate articulated oral responses without thought being given as to how or where they originate.

Articulated speech patterns emerge as they have been learned or programmed. A distorted *S* will come forth distorted, and an omitted R will continue to be omitted in the words in which it should appear. The muscle patterns for the production of the articulated sounds for speech are neurologically programmed and synergically controlled by the cerebellum.

Programs or behaviors that have been learned or programmed can be altered or changed to the extent that the nervous system can be reprogrammed. Then, when the behavior pattern is called for, a new computed resultant will be omitted, or the new behavior will occur. Phases of the desired program, that are alterations of what has gone before, have now been changed to conform to the new program. New or acceptable behaviors must be learned to replace the old or undesirable ones.

Many hypotheses have been designed to promote changes in behaviors, programs, and learning. Laboratory experiments with animals have been the basis for almost all theories advanced. Learning theories have followed the reasoning of such theorists as Pavlov, Konorski, Skinner, Hull, Thorndyke, Gutherie, Wolpe, and many, many others. The stimulus-response-reward procedure is paramount in these systems. One of the basic principles stressed in these theories is reward, or reinforcement, positive and negative. It must be kept in mind that one of the major emphases in this writing is directed toward a learned motor behavior in human speech.

Man has been called the human animal, but he has more cerebral cortex and is capable of high level refined motor skills that are far above what lower animals can and do achieve. The human being is not strictly a stimulus-response-reward organism. He can think and alter his behaviors in self-desired ways or in ways he thinks are acceptable to those in his environment. He may change his behaviors to practically anything he wants them to be, acceptable or not, regardless of the type of reward he may receive for resorting to such behaviors.

For man, a learning philosophy should be based on the neurophysiology of the acquisition of such behaviors as motor skills and other higher level cerebral functions. He cannot be treated as an animal whose upper levels of behavior are mostly fundamental reflexes.

It is often said that humans are victims of habit. Another way of stating it would be that humans are victims of programmed behaviors. The ways they walk, eat, talk, write, etc., are programmed neurophysiological behaviors. Each individual performs the way he does because of what he has stored in the various segments of his computer, his central nervous system, and how he is programmed to use it. The human brain is the greatest computer ever devised and never will be excelled by man's technology.

How best then are changes in human behavior effected? Changes in programs leading to altered computed resultants or behaviors occur more readily if the desired patterns are programmed, stored, or learned rather than being random approximations. Approximations of the desired behaviors can be learned, programmed, and occur as resultants as regularly as any others. Poor behaviors can become habits as easily as good ones. Based on the neurophysiology of learning, one procedure that appears to be essential in learning, changing, or altering motor behaviors is repetition of the desired pattern until it becomes programmed in the nervous system and readily available when requested. Many of the therapies or treatments that are to be suggested require repetition if they are to be used to change the speech behaviors in the person who stutters.

The initial phase of a treatment or therapy program for the establishment of more normal speech for those who have a problem of stuttering should be directed toward the elimination of the symptoms and/or the characteristics of the problem. These symptoms or characteristics have developed into habit patterns and have become accessories to the basic problems of repetitions, hesitations, etc., in the speech of the person who stutters. These deviant behaviors will not be approached in the order in which they tend to appear in the total speaking performance. Each of the basic fundamentals will be presented in a sequence that should lead to the acquisition of more normal speech.

The therapy program to be recommended need not be followed. Some therapists know that what they have to offer the person who stutters is effective and will guide the individual to more normal speech behaviors. A word of caution must be extended concerning the possibility of affording the patient a distraction that will bring about only temporary relief from stuttering. Any therapeutic procedure may be adopted as a distraction if it is given with the suggestion that this will fix or cure his stuttering. Best results are obtained if he is advised that none of the techniques alone, etc., that will be administered will correct the problem of stuttering. Its remediation requires that all of the parts or of the pieces of normal speaking must be correct, in so far as humanly possible, and these facets of speech must be incorporated so as to occur as a total behavior. The person who stutters can and does make a distraction of anything he desires to use if he thinks it will help him.

The therapeutic procedures that follow have been used by this author with very good success. They are offered with the knowledge that they may not prove successful for the therapist or his clients. It all depends on how they are used and how much faith is generated. The patient, the client, or the case will be definitely influenced by confidence displayed for the therapy. The client will have only as much faith and trust in what is being done for him as the therapist has in himself and the program. Thus, administering this program should yield positive results for persons of all ages who have a stuttering problem, regardless of how mild or severe the problem may be.

It was noted in Chapter 4 that the symptoms of stuttering are in fact a syndrome or form a symptom complex. The first symptom that needs to be altered is the excessive muscle tension that is apparent in persons who stutter at all age levels. Human beings always seem to perform skilled motor acts or function better from a relaxed base or point of departure. Relaxation can be accomplished in many ways. There have been many programs recommended that can be used to promote relaxation. There was a time when speech therapy facilities had a relaxation chair or table, but this custom seems to have been abandoned in keeping with current speech correction philosophies.

One notable approach to relaxation was Jacobson's (1953) *Progressive Relaxation*. This program was designed to teach the patient to progressively relax muscles to the extent that minimal muscle tensions could be appreciated and released voluntarily. The program was designed to proceed from the larger to the smaller muscles and thus achieve total relaxation. The program is good, but involved, and takes considerable time to complete. With the person who stutters, time is important, and he tends to be impatient. There are quicker methods available to achieve what is needed in most situations.

Other relaxation programs have been advised. One recommended by Palmer (1951) was said to be that of a Scandinavian masseur and had resulted in an acceptable degree of relaxation. In this procedure the subject is asked to lie down, preferably on a low comfortable table that is sturdy and long enough to accommodate the entire length of the person. (An ideal table is approximately 6 feet, 6 inches in length, and about 2 feet, 2 inches in height, and is padded with foam rubber and covered with vinyl for easy cleaning.) This relaxation procedure starts with the feet and ankles, then progressively includes the shoulders, the hands and arms, the neck, the face and jaw, and finishes with the muscles of respiration. It is possible that the subject may fall asleep while going through this therapy as he becomes more and more relaxed.

In each of the procedures that follow, the therapist, pathologist, or practitioner is assisting by taking the parts of the patient's anatomy through the prescribed movements. The subject is to perform the movements slowly and deliberately and feel the tightening of the muscles as it occurs. He also is to develop an appreciation of the feeling of the relaxed muscles after the movements. After the prescribed pattern with a particular part of the anatomy is completed, the therapist is to take that part through a series of movements passively in order to determine how well the flexor, extensor, rotary, and other muscles have relaxed. Complete relaxation is usually noted when the part can be moved passively without any resistance in any of the motions listed here. These motions are extension, flexion, rotation, abduction, adduction, supination, pronation, etc., as they apply to the particular part of the body being manipulated. A slow, easy pace tends to achieve the best results.

As noted above, this therapy is started with the feet, ankles, and legs. As the subject lies supine on the table he is asked to extend the ankle with the toes pointed away from the body. He is to hold this position while he feels the tension that is present in the ankle and leg in performing this movement. Next he is to relax and return the ankle and foot to a neutral position. He is then to flex the ankle and extend the toes; they are turned up toward the knee, and the leg is held straight. This position is held as before, then relaxed. The subject is asked to turn the foot away from the midline, twisting the knee and leg to the outside, and to hold this position. He next turns the foot to the inside, rotating the knee and leg in the same direction, holding it, then relaxes. The subject is asked to describe a circle with his foot, making sure that it goes the full distance possible in each arc. He is to do this five or six times, then stop and relax. In each of the movements he is to develop an appreciation of the muscle tensions that occur and an awareness of the feeling of relaxed muscles. The other foot and ankle are taken through the same procedure, step by step.

The pattern now changes slightly. The patient is still in the supine position. He is asked to flex his hip and knee with the toes and foot clear of the table. The ankle is extended with the toes pointed away from the body, held, and released. The ankle is next flexed, with the toes pointing toward the knee, held, and released. The foot is made to describe a circle again, with the ankle being turned in every direction to its fullest extent on each segment or arc. The foot and leg are returned to the resting position on the table. The other leg, ankle, and foot repeat the same procedures.

The treatment now shifts to the shoulders. The subject is to move both shoulders up toward his ears and to hold the position. He then releases it. Next the shoulders are pulled down toward the feet, held, and released. The shoulders are then pulled back against the table, as in sticking out the chest, held, and released. Following this, they are pulled forward toward the midline as in starting a self-embrace, but just the shoulders move. This position is held and then released. The shoulders are made to describe a circle, moving together and to the fullest extent possible in each arc. It will be found that many persons who stutter are not able to do this correctly and may need assistance. After going through the circular pattern four to five times, the subject is told to relax.

The hands and forearms are now the point of attention. With the upper arm resting on the table and away from the body about 45 degrees, the elbow is flexed and the forearm is elevated 90 degrees in the air. Next the fingers are clenched, making a fist. The wrist is rotated so that the fist describes a complete circle. This is done several times; then the fist is relaxed, and the fingers are extended and spread wide apart. The fingers are held in this extended position, and again the wrist is rotated several times and relaxed. The forearm is then returned to the table, and the other hand and wrist are taken through the identical procedure.

The arms are placed alongside the trunk, on the table. The hands are supinated, palms up. The subject is to imagine that there is a bar lying across his body at the level of the palms of his hands. This is a very heavy bar, with weights on both ends. The weight suggested can be any that would afford the subject a challenge in lifting it. He is told to grasp the bar with the hands and slowly lift it, very slowly (without bending the elbows). He needs to be reminded repeatedly how heavy it is. This procedure should produce an effect similar to that of isotonic exercises. There should be a tensing of both the agonistic and antagonistic muscles involved in this movement. When the hands are about 6 inches above the level of the body, the subject is told to hold the bar steady at that point for several seconds, then to drop it. The hands and arms fall back to the table and he relaxes.

The program now moves to the neck. The head is pushed back against the table, held, and relaxed. The chin, with the mouth closed, is depressed to the chest, held, and relaxed. The head is made to go in a circle, or rotated several times and then relaxed.

The muscles of the face are now given consideration. The

forehead is wrinkled by elevating the eyebrows. This position should be held and relaxed. The opposite movement is done by pulling the eyebrows down. This process is all done with the frontalis muscle. These two positions or movements are then interchanged several times and stopped. The lips are pursed tightly, held, and relaxed; then a smile is initiated, with the angles of the mouth pulled laterally. These two movements are also interchanged several times and then stopped.

Work with the muscles of respiration concludes this program. The subject's pulse is taken. He is instructed to breathe in while the therapist counts to three, in time with the pulse beat. He then breathes out to the same count and beat. This procedure is repeated several times, with the therapist applying slight resistance to the chest as the subject inhales. He then is advised to continue breathing this way for a few minutes and just relax.

As noted earlier, this relaxation program has been found to be effective with persons who tend to be very tense and who are in need of some relief and relaxation. The total program usually takes about half an hour to do correctly — which, in many instances, is a little too long. This author has devised a shortened version of the program above and has found it to be quite effective. It can be done in a very few minutes, with good levels of relaxation accomplished. The subject also can do this program by himself at home.

The subject is supine, on his back, on a table designed for relaxation. The first few times through the program he will need some assistance, but should be able to perform it by himself shortly thereafter. The individual is instructed to flex or draw his leg up at the hip and flex the knee. The lower leg inclines toward the table, but clear of it. At the same time the foot is pointed up toward the knee as the ankle is flexed. This position is drawn up tightly and held and then relaxed as the leg is returned to the table. Next the leg is lifted off the table and extended. The hip is slightly flexed to accomplish this position, and the foot is elevated about 1 foot above the table. The knee is extended or straightened, and the toes and foot are pointed away from the knee as the ankle is extended. This position is held for a few seconds, then released, and the leg dropped back to the table. These two positions then are interchanged several times: first, forced flexion and then extension of the hip, knee and ankle, or foot. The leg then is released and allowed to drop to the table. Next, the therapist should rotate the leg back and forth at the hip by placing a hand at knee level and moving it slowly. The therapist also should place a hand under the knee and raise it up and down slowly to test the degree of relaxation obtained. There should be no resistance. The same procedures are carried out with the other leg.

The shoulders are maneuvered as outlined in the program previously given. In brief, they are pulled up simultaneously toward the ears, held, and released. Then they are pulled down toward the feet, held, and released. Next, the shoulders are pulled back against the table, held, and released. This procedure is followed by pulling them forward and in toward the midline, holding them for a few seconds, and then returning them to the table. The shoulders then are taken in a circular movement, with the therapist making sure that they travel through the full extent of each arc, and then relaxed. As noted earlier, this process appears to be a difficult maneuver for persons who stutter, and they often need assistance. Upon completion of the circular motion, the therapist should grasp the person's shoulders and move them up and down off the table to assess the amount of remaining tension, if any.

The arms are relaxed in the following manner. The elbow is force-flexed, with the forearm supinated and the fist clenched, as would a boy showing the size of his biceps. This position is maintained for a few seconds, and then the forearm is returned to the table. Next, the arm is fully extended with the forearm pronated, palm down, and the fingers extended and spread wide apart. The arm then is lifted off the table and away from the body at about a 30 degree angle from the shoulder. The position is held for a few seconds then then released. The two positions then are performed interchangeably through four to six repetitions, which end with the arm extended and dropped to the table. Next, the therapist gently grasps the back of the arm, just above the elbow, with the left hand and takes the forearm above the wrist with the right hand. The shoulder, upper arm, and forearm are moved in a circle and other maneuvers to determine the state of relaxation obtained.

The head and neck become involved, with the subject moving the head back against the table, and down to his chest, as in the previously mentioned program. Each of these positions is held for a few seconds, and then the head is returned to the neutral position and the neck and shoulder muscles are relaxed. Two additional movements should be included: the head is turned to the left, chin pointing toward the shoulder, held, and released, and then turned toward the right shoulder in like manner. The head is now rotated through the four positions about four times, then stopped at the normal resting position, with the neck and shoulder muscles relaxed. The therapist takes the chin and gently moves the head back and forth and notes any tensions that may remain.

Next, the facial muscles are approached by wrinkling the forehead and then relaxing it, and thus releasing the contraction of the frontalis muscle. This procedure is followed by pulling the eyebrows down and then releasing the pull of the muscles. These two positions are interchanged several times and discontinued, with relaxation following. The lips are pursed and released. This process is followed with a smile and release. Again the positions are interchanged several times, with relaxation following the cessation of movement.

The muscles of mastication, the jaw muscles, are included in this program. The teeth are clenched and thus create tension in the jaw-closing muscles, and then the bite is released. The jaw, the mandible, is depressed, with the mouth opened against resistance. This action produces tension in the jaw-opening muscle groups, which include the supra– and infrahyoid muscles and associated musculature. This process is repeated several times. Upon cessation, the therapist, and later the subject, places a hand under the chin and moves the jaw rapidly in a series of light movements, which cause clicking of the teeth. This exercise also brings about relaxation of the extrinsic, and possibly the intrinsic, muscles of the larynx.

Imaginary weight lifting also may be used in this program. If is determined that there is tension in the respiratory musculature and further relaxation is indicated, then by all means weight lifting should be used. It is usually found that the subject, after completing the foregoing program, is relaxed.

BREATHING

After the subject is relaxed, the next symptoms or problems that must be corrected are the deviant breathing patterns. It will be recalled that both the quiet and speech breathing patterns of the person who stutters are found to vary widely from those of normal speakers. Quiet, normal breathing is a rhythmic, synchronous pattern that is in phase with the cardiac rhythms. It is not just diaphragmatic breathing, which is inefficient in that it accounts for only 30 to 60 percent of the normal exchange of air in quiet breathing.

Normal quiet breathing occurs when there is no exertion. Breathing requires thoracic, abdominal, and diaphragmatic movements. On inspiration, the taking in of air, the thorax or chest is elevated; it moves outward and upward. The diaphragm is contracted forward and downward. The abdomen protrudes or comes outward. This movement of the abdomen is in direct relationship to the functioning of the diaphragm. The work phase of the diaphragm is contraction, which pulls the muscle sheath down and forward. For the breathing to be efficient, there must be some displacement of the stomach and liver and other abdominal viscera. Such displacement allows the diaphragm to be fully contracted and thus permit its full benefit to be realized in increasing the size of the thoracic cavity. This movement, combined with that of the chest, causes an enlargement of the thoracic cavity, which creates a vacuum or a decompression in the cavity and causes the air to be pulled into the lungs. Expiration or exhalation is brought about by reversing this process and creating pressure on the lungs. Thus, air is forced out of the lungs.

The normal pattern of respiration is synchronized to the

extent that the inspiratory and expiratory movements of the chest, diaphragm, and abdomen occur together, move out to take in air, and move in to push air out, as traced on a polygraph.

These patterns or movements also are synchronized with the cardiac rhythms as measured by the pulse. In normal breathing, inspiration should occur on two or three pulse beats, and expiration also should occur on two or three pulse beats. In order to be synchronized, the person who breathes in on three pulse beats should breathe out on three pulse beats. In keeping with this, the person who breathes in on two beats should breathe out on two beats. The three-in and three-out pattern seems to predominate. When normal quiet breathing patterns are recorded on a polygraph or kymograph record, the tracings describe a sinusoidal curve.

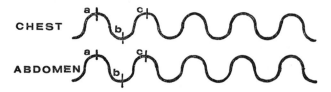

Figure 1: Artist's concept of polygraph tracings depicting movements of chest and abdomen during normal quiet breathing: ab, inspiration; bc, expiration; ac, one respiratory cycle. Curves are parallel.

The tracings indicate inspiration on the downward curvature and expiration on the upward segment of the curve as they illustrate the movements of the chest and abdomen during breathing. For breathing to be normal, these two phases should be close to being identical. Also, the thoracic and abdominal curves should be about the same; the abdominal curve is indicative of diaphragmatic breathing.

Abnormal quiet breathing patterns, as found in persons who stutter, were described in Chapter 4. As a brief review, these abnormal patterns were found to be asynchronous in relation to the cardiac rhythms. There were variations in the length of the inspiratory phase in contrast to that of the expiratory phase of the pattern.

Quite often, the stuttering individual will breathe in on only one pulse beat and breathe out on three or four beats. These respiratory cycles may occur in a series, followed by a period of no breathing, apnea. This period may be succeeded by a deep breath, a pause, and then a return to the asynchronous quiet pattern.

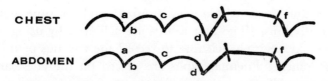

Figure 2: Artist's concept of polygraph tracings depicting movements of chest and abdomen during abnormal quiet breathing: ab, short inspiration; bc, prolonged expiration; ac, one respiratory cycle; de, deep inspiration, expiration; ef, period of no breathing. Curves are often parallel.

The person may have a pattern that is solely diaphragmatic and abdominal.

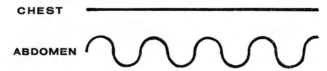

Figure 3: Artist's concept of polygraph tracings depicting an abnormal quiet breathing pattern. The chest is held fixed; the movements of the abdomen indicate only diaphragmatic breathing.

He may have a pattern that is marked with abdominal-thoracic reversals, in which the chest goes one way and the abdomen goes the other throughout the respiratory pattern. Another variation occurs when the individual takes a quick breath in followed by a quick release of air. This process is followed by a period of no breathing; then the pattern is repeated. There also may be a rapid series of quick breaths in and out; then there will be a longer period of apnea before breathing is resumed.

The deviant quiet breathing patterns should and can be

brought within normal limits by therapeutic procedures. Palmer (1951) and his medical staff devised a technique that tends to alter these deviant patterns, a program called block breathing. The physiological and metabolic aspects of this program will not be discussed here, but they are relevant.

If block breathing is carried out as designed and occurs periodically, there should be a change in the respiratory patterns so that they become more sychronized and in tune with the cardiac rhythms. The best results are achieved by using a polygraph or kymograph machine to record the tracings of the chest and abdomen. Pneumographs are placed on the chest and abdomen in order to record their movements. The tracings recorded should resemble a box without a lid and then a box turned upside down.

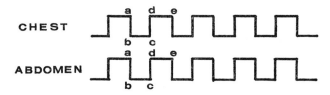

Figure 4: Artist's concept of polygraph tracings depicting therapeutic block breathing for correcting quiet breathing. Chest and abdomen move together: ab, quick inspiration; bc, no breathing; cd, quick expiration; de, no breathing.

The subject may be sitting, or lying in a supine position. He is instructed to take in a breath as rapidly as possible, then hold it, and not release or take in any air until he is told to do so. Then he is to release the air as rapidly as possible, stop, and neither release nor take in any air until he is told to do so. The pattern then is repeated eight to ten times. This is all done to a count established by taking the pulse. This author has achieved the best results by using a 4:4 pattern.

Also, the subject must adhere to the following sequence: breathe in, hold it, three, four; breathe out, hold it, three, four. The count is with the pulse beat. The therapist must direct the pattern and count the sequence. This sequence can be shortened to in, hold it, three, four; out, hold it, three, four. This action must be done voluntarily by the subject, and he must cooperate fully if the faulty quiet breathing patterns are to be changed.

After repeating the block pattern eight to ten times, the subject is told to relax. There will be a period of apnea, no breathing. This will be followed by a deep breath. Then there should be a rhythmical and synchronized quiet breathing pattern with three pulse beats in and three pulse beats out. The polygraph tracings now should reflect dual sinusoidal curves, one for thoracic and the other for abdominal movement. A well-practiced and experienced pathologist can detect these movements with his hands; to acquire this skill takes years of experience using the visible polygraph tracings as a guide.

The normal quiet breathing should continue for a period of time before there is a relapse and the individual returns to his old breathing pattern. Some persons change over to the new pattern readily after a few therapy sessions; others take a longer period of time, and may require many therapy sessions over a period of several months. The majority of those receiving this breathing program do change their quiet breathing pattern to one that is more acceptable. The program should be continued until a permanent pattern is established. The subject is usually able to practice this program on his own after a few sessions — which should expedite the formation of the desired behavior.

This breathing program appears to bring about oxygen–carbon dioxide changes and metabolic changes that are within acceptable limits for the organism, to the extent that it results in improved quiet breathing in the majority of subjects. There will be some subjects who do not readily alter their patterns. This slowness may be due to a lack of cooperation or physiological problems that preclude any alterations of their breathing behaviors. If the program is presented correctly, all subjects should improve and be better for having done so. This program is not a cure for stuttering, but is a revision of one of the symptoms and a necessary step toward developing normal breathing for speech. The subject must be reminded that this program will not correct his stuttering, but rather improve his faulty quiet breathing patterns.

On each respiratory cycle, normally, 500 cubic centimeters of air are exchanged by inhaling and exhaling. This fact is mentioned because some individuals who stutter have a low vital capacity. Low vital capacity is commonly found in persons who have certain diseases or have suffered a stroke, etc. This does not mean that persons who stutter have a disease or have had a stroke. Vital capacity is measured as the total amount of air that can be expelled after the lungs have been fully expanded by the deepest possible breath. Measured by the metric system, vital capacity is said to be about 4.5 liters. According to Howell (1949), the vital capacity of an average male, in liters, should be two and one-half times his body surface area measured in square meters. The female tends to have slightly lower vital capacity, that is, two times her body surface area measured in square meters.

For speech, it is noted that an individual should have a vital capacity that will permit him to produce a prolonged, moderately loud *ah* for fifteen seconds. Some persons who stutter can hold the *ah* for only five or six seconds. These people consistently run out of breath while trying to speak; they are forever gasping for air, or trying to force out air that is not readily available for speech. The acquisition of normal quiet breathing tends to aid in solving this problem, but it is often necessary to work directly on increasing the vital capacity.

After a good start toward correcting the quiet breathing patterns is achieved, correction of deviant speech breathing practices should be initiated. Persons who stutter have a variety of divergent breathing patterns for speech when compared to persons with fluent speaking habits. Exhaled air is the source of energy or power for speech. If the production of this energy is defective, it will contribute to imperfections in the final output, speech.

The speech breathing patterns of fluent speakers follow a definite sequence. First, there is inhalation of air, which occurs rather quickly, but not so rapidly as the inspiration in block breathing. The tracing for this phase in speech breathing, as seen on a polygraph, is downward and at an angle of about 20 to 30 degrees from the horizontal lines; this position will vary slightly.

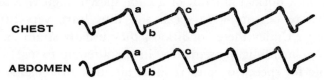

Figure 5: Artist's concept of polygraph tracings depicting normal speech breathing patterns: ab, inspiration; bc, expiration while speaking; a, release of leftover air and reversal of breathing musculature; b, reversal of breathing musculature and release of preparatory air for speech.

At the end of inhalation, there is a reversal of the respiratory musculature and a limited release of air. This action is indicated in the tracings as a small arc. At this point the individual initiates speech, which can continue for a period of time, depending on what is to be said and the depth of his vital capacity for speaking. This flow of air for speech output is represented in Figure 5 as a diagonal line extended up and to the right from the reversing arc.

A speaker usually does not exhaust his air supply, but takes a breath at a convenient place in his verbal discourse, where punctuation may occur, and at a point before which exertion is necessary to continue the flow of speech. As he prepares to inhale, there is again a release of air and a reversal of the respiratory musculature as the inspiratory phase occurs. This process is shown in the polygraph tracing as a small arc that leads into the downward trace of inhalation.

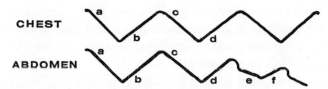

Figure 6: Artist's concept of polygraph tracings depicting a defective speech breathing pattern noted in some persons who stutter: ab, inspiration; bc, expiration while speaking; c, absence of release of leftover air and reversal of breathing musculature and release of preparatory air for speech; ef, abdominal reversal to chest pattern.

Individuals who stutter seem to have a variety of deviations in their speech breathing patterns. There are those who tend to take in a normal amount of air for speech, then release most of it before beginning to speak and thus leave very little for speaking. Under these conditions, they usually strain and contract the breathing musculature in an attempt to use air not available for speech output, residual air; this air remains in the lungs and cannot be exhaled. This process results in gasping for air in the attempt to continue speaking. The length of response in a given breathing cycle will vary, depending on the amount of air inhaled on the inspiratory gasp.

Another problem that is noticeable in the speech breathing patterns of persons who stutter is found at the end of the inspiratory phase. Instead of there being a normal reversal of the respiratory musculature with a slight release of air, as indicated by the small arc in the polygraph tracings (Fig. 6), there is a point of departure indicating that the individual is attempting to initiate speech at precisely the moment that he begins to exhale, and is abruptly reversing the respiratory musculature from inspiration to expiration (Fig. 6).

At the termination of the exhalation of the flow of air for speaking, the person who stutterers does not have a normal release of air and reversal of the respiratory muscles for inhalation. Again in the tracings, this terminal point is indicated by a sharp reversal of the musculature, as for a gasp of air. This pattern tends to be quite common (Fig. 6).

The stuttering individual may have speech breathing patterns during which he holds his chest in a fixed position and talks only with diaphragmatic breathing. This would be depicted in the polygraph tracings as a continuous horizontal line, while the abdominal movements would be shown as a speech breathing pattern similar to those noted above.

The person may have a breathing pattern for speaking in which the thoracic movements are in one direction and the abdominal movements in the opposite direction. In this action the chest is being depressed as an ascending speech line (Fig. 7), but at the same time the abdomen is being pushed out or extended. The tracings that indicate faulty abdominal movements would be either a straight line or the reverse of those for the chest.

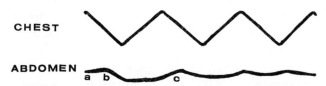

Figure 7: Artist's concept of polygraph tracings depicting a defective speech breathing pattern noted in some persons who stutter. Chest curve reveals defective speech breathing: abdomen moves very little and is in opposition to chest movements. (Thoracic-abdominal reversals.)

During the exhalation phase of breathing for speech, individuals who stutter, regardless of age, resort to inspiratory gasps that interrupt the steady flow of air exhaled for speech. These are noted on the polygraph as small reversals or changes in the outflow of air while speaking (Fig. 8). These may occur with a block of some type, or as short inspiratory gasps taken in an attempt to continue the flow of exhaled air.

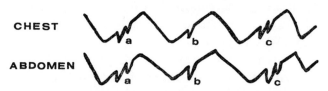

Figure 8: Artist's concept of polygraph tracings depicting a defective speech breathing pattern noted in some persons who stutter: a, b, and c. inspiratory gasps during expiration for speech.

In view of the many varieties and deviations noted in speech breathing patterns of persons who stutter, it undoubtedly appears that it is unlikely that much can be done to restore or change these patterns to conform more closely to those considered to be normal or acceptable. This notion, however, is not the case. These patterns are subject to change, as are quiet breathing patterns through the use of specific therapeutic techniques.

In order to obtain breathing patterns for speech that resemble or closely approximate those of fluent speakers, the subject must be directed in ways that facilitate this mode of behavior. The basic form of the desired pattern must be kept in mind by the therapist at all times (Fig. 5). The intake and release of breath must be coordinated so that the chest and abdomen and the diaphragm (the same movement as the abdomen) move together. This coordination should be the first phase to be established.

The inhalation and exhalation of air with abdominal and thoracic coordination should have already begun through the work done on quiet breathing. It will be recalled that the establishment of normal quiet respiration should constitute the first phase in the achievement of acceptable breathing behaviors. If this respiration has been initiated and improvement is noted, the development of an acceptable speech breathing pattern is made much easier.

If inhalation can be accomplished with synchronized movement of the respiratory muscles, the subject should be instructed to do so. This action is followed by a somewhat forced exhalation in the form of a moderately loud whispered *ah*. The subject should release the air in a slow, prolonged manner. This expulsion of air should continue as long as the flow is easy and the coordinated depression of the chest and abdomen is maintained. The flow of air must not be forced; it must be stopped when it appears that the contrary is taking place. The duration of this pattern may be limited at first as quite often there is an abdominal reversal. The abdomen will begin to protrude, particularly as the subject approaches the end of the easy flow of air. When this protrusion occurs, the subject should stop the exhalation of air and relax.

Another breath is taken and released slowly and evenly as a moderately loud whispered *ah*. If the abdomen begins to protrude, and the subject is an adolescent or adult, the therapist should suggest to him that the stomach must not come out. It must be explained that the chest and the abdomen must be depressed simultaneously and that this action continues throughout the release of air. If the subject is a child, light pressure or a push on the abdomen may keep it moving in the desired direction. This process also may be used with the adolescent or adult as an aid to the suggestions given. This phase of the program should be repeated until it can be done easily, consistently, and voluntarily without assistance.

When the subject can prolong the whispered *ah* consistently, he is asked to repeat the inhalation and exhalation patterns. This time he is to add another component, phonation, and make a prolonged, voiced, or phonated *ah*. He is to maintain the *ah* as long as it is produced easily and there are no reversals. It may be necessary to alternate back and forth between the whispered *ah* until the transition is made to the voiced *ah* with synchronized thoracic-abdominal movements.

The next step in this program to assist in the development of more normal speech breathing patterns is to have the subject gradually and easily add more rote syllables to the prolonged air stream, inhale, begin the air flow, and say *ah*. To this syllable he should begin to add numbers, slowly, one at a time. He is to extend the *ah* and proceed to add the number *one* in a rather drawn-out manner. He repeats this process, using the same speech breathing patterns, with *ah, one, two,* and then building to *ah, one, two, three, four.* The subject must continue to maintain synchronized breathing and remain relaxed throughout this phase of therapy. If there is a breakdown in the breathing patterns, the program must be regressed, or taken back a step or two. Normal speech breathing must be achieved at the lower level and then gradually brought back to the level where the problem occurred. If the therapy is successful to the extent that the counting can be done repeatedly with sound breathing patterns, the next step is introduced.

Now the basic breathing for speech is in the process of being developed. The next procedure is an extension of the pattern immediately completed. The subject is asked to take a breath and count from one to four. Then he releases whatever air he may have left over. Another breath is taken, and he counts from one to five, and releases leftover air. Next he takes another breath with a count of one to six; another breath with a count of one to seven; and then one more, with a count of one to eight. After the last number in each series, the subject is to release what air is leftover, if any, take another breath, and count the next series. The counting is done slowly. It is best if done to the beat of the pulse. This coordination helps establish a rhythm and rate that is in keeping with his basic cardiac and physiological rhythms. At times there appears to be a fast and a slow phase to the pulse beat. When this action seems to occur, the slower beat should be the one to consider.

The series counting should continue from one to four, progressively, up to and including *one* to *eight,* until the breathing and counting are consistent and easily performed. This action may not take long to accomplish in that these patterns are more in keeping with normal respiration and the subject's basic rhythm for speaking.

One more modification of the speech breathing patterns needs to be made before they duplicate those of the fluent speaker. This is the release of air, after inhalation, just before starting the outflow for speaking. The individual should be requested to release a little air as he starts to count the series. This should be in the form of an unaccented *h,* or an easy starting of the flow of air. This release of air should not be stopped and another started before speaking. The subject must continue the *h* or release of air into his speech, or, as in this instance, count. He must be advised not to focus his attention on this aspect and use it as a distraction.

Throughout the therapy for breathing, the person who stutters must be reminded that the change in breathing patterns will not correct his stuttering. He is merely working on one of the problems of the symptom complex. All the symptoms of the complex must be corrected, or eliminated, before he can expect to develop the type of fluent speech he desires. Continued care must be taken to make sure that this person does not use breathing as a distraction. If he does, the desired effect of change to normal speech breathing will be lost and will suffer the consequences of all distractions.

The subject now should be able to use without difficulty this replica of what the fluent speaker does with his speech breathing. The next transition is from series counting to another rote speaking behavior, saying nursery rhymes. The selected nursery rhyme for making this change is "One, two, buckle my shoe." A breath is to be taken before saying each line. The subject should release some air as he begins each line, as above. At the end of each line, whatever air is leftover is released. Another breath is taken to start the second line, and whatever air is leftover at the end of that line is released. This breathing sequence is repeated line after line. Now the subject is using the breathing and speaking patterns as he did in series of counting from one to four up to one to eight.

Further extensions of the breathing pattern and speaking now can be made. The individual should extend the single exhalation of air so that he is now able to say two lines before releasing the leftover air and taking another breath to say two more lines, etc. Other nursery rhymes, days of the week, and material spoken by rote are to be added at this time. Care must be taken that the subject continues to use the proper speech breathing patterns as he progresses through the different materials. The person who stutters now is being afforded the opportunity to speak fluently and use normal speech breathing patterns.

In order to learn the mechanics of normal speech and feed them back into the nervous system so that new programs can be established and stored, the person who stutters must be provided with the wherewithal to do so, fluent speech. One must be constantly mindful of the fact that motor behaviors are learned as they are fed back into the nervous system. If normal or acceptable motor programs are to be accessible on demand, they must be learned, stored, and made as computed resultants from the cerebellum in the desired form. The emphasis at this time is still on changing the deviant symptoms and/or characteristics of stuttering, and providing the person who stutters with more normal behaviors as replacements.

Thus far in the program the materials for practice have been what are commonly referred to as "by rote." These materials are information that has been memorized to the extent that it can be spoken without thinking. It just "comes out" when requested. It seems that much information given in daily conversations is by rote. It all has been memorized quite well. It may be stated that the materials used for practice thus far have been low in propositional value and, therefore, are spoken without the need to think ahead and give thought to what is to be said. Some persons who stutter have difficulty even when this rote level of material is suggested. In such instances it may be necessary to provide materials that are on a lower propositional level than these. In some cases, redundancy of the material produces familiarity to the extent that the thinking-ahead behavior is reduced or eliminated. Call it adaptation, if desired.

There is now the need to introduce higher levels of propositional interchange of communication. Questions and answers should be initiated. The questions are to be directed toward responses or answers that can be given by rote, information that has been memorized and can be repeated without thinking. The questions are asked by the therapist. The answers are to be given in complete sentences by the subject. During this exchange, the subject must continue to use the speech breathing patterns already learned and remain relaxed.

There may be a question in some readers' minds as to the "roteness" of the information asked for in this question-and-answer interaction. What, however, could be more "by rote" than asking a person, What is your name? Where do you live? What is your address? What is your telephone number? Where do you work? Where do you go to school? In what city do you live? Do you have any brothers and sisters? What are their names? The answers to these questions have been memorized and should be forthcoming without requiring thought.

From the rote material, the propositional level is gradually increased until the subject can carry on a fairly fluent conversation. Why "fairly fluent"? Only fairly fluent because the therapist is dealing only with some of the characteristics of the problem, and there are more. It is at this phase of the program that increased difficulty will be encountered because the problem of thinking ahead may become more apparent.

At this point, also, it will be necessary to reiterate the processes of normal speaking behavior. Attention will have to be drawn to the normal procedure of thinking out loud. The subject will have to become more aware of what happens to his thinking process when rote materials are spoken, and develop a feeling for this type of performance. This information is expounded on later in this chapter.

ARTICULATION OF SPEECH

The person who stutters is being directed through a program from which should evolve more fluent speech output. The actual movements for the articulation of speech are coordinated muscle behaviors that are organized in a time scheme in such a way as to modify a phonated or nonphonated air stream. These organized patterns result in words. The basic single component or sound in each word is a noise. This concept should be explained to the stuttering individual.

Speech is an assortment of puffs, hisses, and other noises. Except in a few instances, these noises or sounds carry absolutely no meaning in and of themselves. An *S* is a hiss; a *P* is a puff of air, etc. The vowels are noises that are voiced and consist of *A, E, I, O, U,* with some modifications of each occurring to lengthen or shorten them. There are also some voiced consonants. Isolated noises that tend to carry meaning are *SH* for quieting, *M* and *U* for satisfaction, *O* for surprise or a question. There are probably others, but these are samples.

It should be pointed out to the person who stutters that the sound on which he has a tendency to stutter is just a noise, one that he can make anytime in isolated form without any difficulty. Since he is quite capable of making the noise, there is no need for him to avoid making it.

During the course of therapy, it is often desirable to have the subject prepare sentences using all of the speech phonemes. It is suggested that individual assignments be given for each of the speech sounds. The subject should be encouraged to use the sound assigned in as many words as possible in one sentence.

The first word of each sentence should have the sound as the first letter. In the therapy situation, the sentences should be read aloud. Special emphasis is to be placed on the melody, rhythm, and accent patterns used in each sentence and on multi-syllable words. This practice develops an acquaintance with the sounds of speech, the accent patterns used in normal speaking, and the variations used in melody. It should be pointed out that melody, rhythm, and accent patterns are important in speaking. Variations in these patterns also produce differences in the meaning of what is being said.

RATE OF SPEECH

As noted in Chapter 4, persons who stutter tend to have problems with rapid speech output. This difficulty may not be a constant pattern, but appears to occur spasmodically. There is a tendency to rush ahead in speaking when the possibility of fluent speech is apparent. This rushing usually terminates in a block, unless the speaker terminates his speaking before the block occurs. This is not cluttering.

Work on the rate of speech output may be indicated when the individual is unable to adapt to the rote behavior rates presented. It may be necessary to work deliberately at slowing down his rate to one that is in keeping with his physiological rhythms and capabilities. Telling him to slow down will not accomplish the desired results.

The rate of speech should be within acceptable limits for the age and general physiology of the individual. The best guide available for setting this rate is the cardiac rhythm or the pulse.

Speech is a rhythmical, melodic behavior. All speech patterns are marked with melody, rhythm, and accent. The nature of these three elements is as semantically important as the words chosen to express oneself. How something is spoken is as important in conveying the desired meaning of the message as are the words used. Alterations in melody, rhythm, or accent can change the simplest utterance from meaning one thing to meaning something entirely different. Children are greatly affected by the manner in which things are said to them, and this reaction is altered only slightly with maturity as the meanings of words gain more importance as carriers of information. As an example: "Your words say you love me, but the way you say it leaves doubt in my mind."

As noted above, speech is marked with melody, rhythm, and accent patterns. These elements also play an important part in controlling the rate of speaking. The melody of a response tends to follow the rhythm and accent. The more heavily accented syllables in a word, or particular words in a phrase or sentence, receive the melodic changes in voice. The flow of syllables in isolated words and words in sentences, with their accented and unaccented segments, gives rise to the rhythm of what is said. Good normal speech is not uttered in a monotonous monotone; it is melodic, rhythmic, and alive.

In using these elements of speech to control the rate of speaking, the subject is directed in the following manner. In rote materials, he is to tap the finger or the hand to the pulse beat to the accented syllables and words, such as in "Ońe, twó, búckle my shóe." There the ' indicates those words or syllables in words that are to receive an accent. This procedure can be carried on into prepared sentences, as noted in the section on articulation above. An accented syllable or word is to be marked with an ' and then spoken in the same manner. Rhythm and melody appear to "fall into place" if this accenting is done correctly.

Other gross motor actions can be incorporated to aid in this endeavor. Clapping the hands, walking to the beat, etc., can be of benefit. After establishing good melody, rhythm, and accent patterns with gross motor acts, the person should duplicate the spoken passage without a gross motor act. He should begin to develop a feeling for these patterns and adapt them to his speaking behavior. Thus, he gains some control of his rate of speech. This process must not be allowed to become a distraction. The melody, rhythm, and accent patterns must be within normal limits and not exaggerated. This therapy is yet another step in the acquisition of more normal speech. The therapist should be certain that he understands this fact.

READING

Another form of communication needs to be explained: reading. It should be pointed out that written words are graphic or printed symbols of what a person says. They mean that someone has taken the time to gather what he wanted to say and put it down on paper. When these printed or written words are read aloud, they are converted into oral speech. Oral communication appears to have preceded the written or graphic forms of communication. This is true in every language. Languages differ only in the sounds or phonemes used and their time scheme. Words are written with different symbols, but blue is blue regardless of the word used for saying it or the symbols used to write it down.

As the person in therapy becomes more fluent in speaking, reading should be included in the therapy program to assist him in developing this additional form of communication, which he will use periodically. The acquisition of fluent reading will contribute to his overall improved communicative behavior.

SECONDARY SYMPTOMS

Thus far in the treatment program designed to reduce or change the symptoms of stuttering, the person has been relaxed and aided in developing quiet breathing patterns. He also has worked toward developing normal speech breathing patterns. Practice on more normal speech has been realized by way of rote materials. Somewhere along the way, consideration must be given to the secondary symptoms he has developed. It will be recalled that secondary symptoms tend to be those devices and behaviors to which the person who stutters has resorted in his attempts to relieve his stuttering. These are no longer of any benefit to him. They are an added burden and make his problem appear worse.

When these accessory behaviors are attacked during therapy, the subject should be informed as to what they are and how they came to develop. He must be convinced that they are superfluous behaviors and not a part of his initial problem. His adding them to his already disturbing problem makes it seem worse. He must be advised to forget them and not to resort to them ever again. In some cases, suggestion is sufficient to bring about a reduction in the use of distractions; other subjects may need further assistance in order to eliminate their secondary symp- *//* toms.

In those instances where suggestion does not satisfactorily relieve the symptoms, further measures will be needed. Some persons who stutter are quite unaware of what they do while speaking. It may be necessary to point out each secondary symptom as it occurs and expose it for what it is, an added useless behavior. With still others, it may be necessary to have them observe themselves in a mirror and note what they are doing and again point out the needless accessory behavior.

If the symptoms persist, then negative practice is a good approach to use. In this, the subject voluntarily performs the act or behavior he wishes to change in front of a mirror. He does so over and over again, while speaking, until the undesirable trait is abandoned. The symptom now becomes an activity to be avoided because the individual has become saturated and disgusted with it. Many undesirable motor behaviors can be eliminated in this manner.

One secondary symptom that appears to be exceptionally difficult to eliminate is the subject's chronic pattern of looking away or averting the eyes and head while speaking; particularly when he "sees" a block approaching. The answer sounds simple, but it is not. A remission of this behavior may be slowly accomplished by having the individual look at the person to whom he is speaking. It is not necessary to look the other person in the eye; this direction would raise the propositionality of the encounter. The subject may pick out several different places to look: the hairline, the nose, the mouth, the ear, or the face in general. He is to maintain this eye contact while speaking. If he starts to look away during therapy sessions, the therapist either should tell him, or indicate by a signal, that he must reestablish eye contact. In time, the subject will learn to keep eye contact with the listener and feel more at ease in doing so.

THINKING ALOUD

Most of the symptoms that occur during stuttering now have been considered, and treatment to modify them has been advanced. Finally it is necessary to work at eliminating the true cause for the continuation of stuttering after it should have disappeared as the nervous system grew, developed, and matured.

The problem of extreme importance is the learned behavior of thinking ahead to determine what is to be said while attempting to continue speaking at the same time. This problem was explained in detail in Chapter 5.

When the therapist worked on speech breathing, the subject was introduced to the normal human behavior of speaking without thinking. It had to be explained to him that, in the normal process of thinking-to-speaking, the behavior is more like thinking out loud. Thinking is occurring, but the time interval between the thought and the speech is so rapid that it cannot be appreciated. The process is like "talking off the top of the head." From a practical standpoint, it is thinking out loud.

Thus, the stuttering individual is advised of what he has been doing. Almost all persons who stutter will admit that they do think ahead. A five– or six-year-old child will admit to doing it as readily as an adolescent or an adult. When told of this, one of the standard replies is "How did you know that?"

The subject must be taught that what he is doing is incorrect. He must understand that fact. This thought pattern is the procedure that is getting him into difficulty. With the adolescent and the adult, the therapist can be very specific about this faulty procedure. With the small child, it is best to suggest that he "talk off the top of his head." He is to *do* as he does when counting and saying nursery rhymes. The key phrase to be remembered by the person who is receiving therapy is "Don't think, just talk." Children and adolescents pick up the motto or key phrase quickly. They work at following it faithfully. This attitude is one of the basic reasons why these age groups respond better to therapy than do adults. The other reasons are that the problem behaviors have not become so thoroughly established, and the less mature nervous systems are more amenable to change.

Adults admit to the fact that they think ahead. They say that they try not to do so, but they just do. These deviant patterns in the adult have been thoroughly learned and have become established habits. In his thinking ahead, the adult also has developed an awareness of the sounds and words with which he has trouble. He looks for these as he thinks ahead and anticipates stuttering on them. Now he has compounded the problem. His thinking ahead is disrupting the normal flow of thought-to-speech, and he has added the set pattern of looking for trouble.

The act of looking ahead for trouble sounds and words in speech is one of the reasons for the development of secondary symptoms. These symptoms occur immediately prior to the block or stuttering. The person sees the troubling situation coming and tries to avoid it. He attempts to use a distraction to get through it. These distractions become secondary symptoms. Thus, the adult has a double problem to eliminate as he strives to achieve "Don't think, just talk."

Thinking ahead is a very difficult behavior to eradicate. It can be accomplished with patience, understanding, and use of the treatment program presented. Slowly, but surely, the negative habits can be eliminated, and positive, acceptable speaking behaviors established in their place.

There has been found a procedure that appears to be beneficial in teaching the adolescent and adult temporarily to stop thinking ahead and approximate closely the desired behavior. This procedure requires the person to think first of what he wants to say and then say it. It takes only a second or two to think of the desired response. When the person makes this response, there is no thinking ahead, and the speech is devoid of stuttering patterns, if performed properly. This procedure is not to be used as a distraction or a crutch. It is merely a way of establishing an appreciation for the way the subject should feel when the thought-to-speaking process is performed correctly.

EXTENDING PROPOSITIONAL LEVELS

After the person who stutters has developed fluent speech in the training facility, a propositional hierarchy must be drawn up. This hierarchy is an outline of those situations in which the individual has progressively increasing difficulty with his speech. These events will progress from speaking with the therapist in the therapy room, adding another person to these sessions, and so forth, until the most difficult state of affairs the person must endure is added to the top of the list. It must be remembered that the propositionality of an incident is determined by the person himself. It depends on the value he places on that given circumstance. However, what may be a passable level of propositionality of an incident is determined by the person himself. It depends on the value he places on that speaking situation. Therefore, what may be a moderate level of propositionality for one person may be either higher or lower for another.

Circumstances to be considered are those encountered in social, business, school, family, and other activities. The adult, or adolescent usually can tell in what situations he has greater or less difficulty. These situations should be outlined. The telephone, "the little black monster," always seems to be high in each stutterer's hierarchy.

Once the progressive levels of propositionality have been established, the program should shift slowly so as to begin at the bottom or lower level of the hierarchy and work up. This procedure is very important for the adolescent and the adult. Children tend to generalize their speaking behaviors more easily. They do this without analyzing each situation and preparing themselves to meet it. Older children, adolescents, and adults will vary widely in the preparation needed to carry their newfound fluent speech into these conditions. The basic problem is the recall of what has gone before. The tendency is always to revert to the old habit of thinking ahead, for fear of having trouble; this thinking is precisely the thing that caused the difficulty the previous time and many earlier times.

Each proposed new encounter should be analyzed thoroughly.

Questions should be answered concerning why stuttering occurred in previous endeavors. New attitudes will have to be developed. Rehearsals of the adventure to come and speech that may be exchanged may be needed.

It is beneficial for the therapist to accompany the subject through some of these encounters. Where this action is impossible, the individual should venture out on his own with the suggestion that he can handle it easily if he just remembers what he has learned and follows "Don't think, just talk." Then he is to report on how he handled the situation and what occurred. He is to assess how well he spoke. If trouble arose, what did he do that he should or should not have done? Gradually, he will gain confidence and be able to speak fluently under more and more circumstances. How far he goes depends on himself now. He will need guidance and support for a long time until he is confident that he can be as fluent as the next person.

NORMAL FLUENCY AND NONFLUENCY

During the course of training or therapy, it should be brought to the attention of the person who stutters that no one has fluent, perfect speech at all times. His attention must be directed toward a few facts. The so-called normal or fluent speakers occasionally will "stub their toe." Most people have repetitions, hesitations, prolongations, etc., in their speech. These individuals, however, pay little attention to these occurrences and continue to speak without making an issue of the mishap; or they make some offhand remark and brush it off laughingly. Public speakers may make mistakes and have an occasional interruption in their speech.

There are times when fluent person's speech will deteriorate almost completely. These human beings also are victims of the propositionality of situations in which they find themselves. These situations are often passed off as stage fright. These persons place premiums or values on events in which they must perform. They become speechless, or nearly so, when they face a television camera. They develop a loss for words when they have to talk to the boss. They can become unnerved and speak at such a rapid rate that they are not understood when on the witness stand in court. They may become unable to speak when they attempt to talk to someone for whom they have great admiration.

Normal, fluent speech is not fluent at all times, but it is considered to be normal if it is fluent in most situations and most of the time. Normally, fluent speakers do not make an issue of the problems they have. They merely consider the circumstances, pass off the mishap as "just one of those things," and continue to behave and speak in their usual manner. Persons who stutter do not take their speaking troubles so lightly. One mishap fosters another and creates another crisis when the next similar speaking event is encountered. The subject needs to be informed about such phenomena.

EMOTIONS

Many references have been made to the emotional or psychological problems of the person who stutters. There are authorities who suggest that the cause of stuttering is psychologically or psychoneurotically based. According to the knowledge of this author, however, there have not been personality profiles published that would definitely support these assumptions. Studies that have been done reveal little difference between the persons who stutter and those persons used as controls.

The question arises: Do individuals who stutter have emotional problems as the result of their speaking difficulties? The answer is yes. The emotional aspects are caused by the stuttering problem, but are not the source of the stuttering. Most of these persons are concerned about the problem that prevents them from communicating normally. This concern, however, does not seem to be any greater than that held by other persons who have other types of handicaps. At times, the concern does not show on the surface. Persons with problems try to do the best they can with what they have. Some persons, however, as is a custom with human beings, retreat from situations in which they are fearful of being inadequate. Some individuals lack the confidence necessary to move into society and become contributing members.

On the other hand, there are those who stutter and continue to pursue normal lives and show no fear of any events they may experience. There are a few persons who attempt to overcompensate for their speech problem and become highly aggressive and extroverted.

Whichever route is taken, there are emotional aspects present. Persons who need to have their confidence bolstered should achieve this feeling of assurance as their fluent speech is carried into the many life experiences with which they will come to grips. Encouragement, and successful speaking experiences, should and do tend to alleviate the emotional aspects of the problem of stuttering.

The normalization of all behaviors that contribute to normal speech must be the ultimate goal if the problem is to be corrected.

POSTSCRIPT

In this chapter it has been the objective of the author to present a progressive program designed to restore those basic behaviors that are necessary for the establishment of more normal speech. The therapy suggested has followed a set pattern to lead the therapist or person assisting the stutterer from basic foundations of speech to output of fluent speech.

It must be noted that this is a suggested program, aimed toward best results. Other therapeutic techniques may be attempted and used advantageously. Conditioning, behavior modification techniques, etc., may be beneficial in some instances. Other methods for promoting relaxation and normal breathing patterns may be helpful. The goal of any therapeutic program for the person who stutters must be the establishment of more normal fundamental behaviors that are the basis for fluent speech. How this is achieved, by necessity, will vary from person to person. In some instances, implementation will require modification of the therapies recommended here.

The differences between a program for a child who stutters

and one for an adolescent or adult are, basically, variations in approach. While older persons who stutter can be dealt with openly and directly, a child needs a program that is discreet and subtle. The reasons for his attending the therapy sessions should include something other than his stuttering. Most children have other speech problems; some are very minor while others are more severe. They may have an articulatory disorder and mispronounce particular speech sounds in one way or another. If there is not another speech problem, it may be necessary to create an acceptable reason for his coming to see the therapist.

All of the therapies suggested for the development of normal speaking habits should be administered. Depending upon the age of the child, modifications will need to be considered, with a less direct approach being used with the younger child. Gradually he can be trained to use this idea: "Don't think, just talk." More information concerning the childhood problem of stuttering will be given in Chapter 7.

All individuals who stutter are not going to realize normal, fluent speech as the result of this program, but all should improve markedly. With some, there will be such deep-seated habits that they will be changed only slightly. Yet, there should be change enough so as to be noticeable in their speaking behaviors. With others, there may be defiance, or a strong desire to continue to stutter for some deep-seated reason. In these individuals, stuttering is a convenience that enables them to do things and receive considerations that they feel they could not otherwise realize. They may feel that there are advantages to stuttering. Finally, there will be persons who have the conviction that they will never speak fluently, and who, because of a pessimistic attitude, will refuse to try to correct their problems.

In all of the foregoing procedures, it will be necessary to be patient, to make helpful suggestions, and to allow the subject to have the experience of normal, fluent speech. Experience is an excellent teacher and can change many opinions, beliefs, and behaviors. This process can work in two ways. Repeated failures will facilitate pessimism while successes can promote optimism and the desire to do better.

Summary

This chapter has presented a program designed to relieve the symptoms and characteristics of stuttering. Each symptom has been given consideration and therapy recommended to bring that particular behavior within normal limits. The symptoms of concern are those variations or deviations that have developed in those behaviors rudimentary to fluent speaking, as the result of the neurophysiological variation that is stuttering.

Areas of concern have included hypertonus and defective quiet and speech breathing patterns. Fluent speech is gained through utilizing rote materials that do not require thinking as such. These rote practice elements are used to feed desired patterns into the nervous system. Thought-to-speech behavior is changed in order to eliminate the problem of thinking ahead that brings about the undesirable nervous system conflict and the resultant behavior, stuttering.

A program for dealing with propositional variations was suggested. Therapeutic remission of secondary symptoms was given consideration. Emotional problems were recognized. The muscle acivities involved in the articulation of speech were discussed. Reading, as a form of communication, was noted as a graphic form of oral communication.

The therapy program presented has not been offered as the final word for the remission of stuttering. It is a new look at the rehabilitation of stuttering and the problems associated with it.

Chapter 7

MAINTENANCE OF ESTABLISHED NORMAL COMMUNICATION AND ETC.

THE MAINTENANCE of any newly learned motor behavior by human beings always has posed a problem. After learning a new, acceptable behavior, too often there is regression to the old habit. The human being tends to take the way of least resistance. The improved behavior relapses as a result of failure to continue to work at making it as much of a habit as was the unwanted behavior. A person needs continued encouragement and assistance to perpetuate the new habit.

The person who stutters has the same problem. It is easy for him to regress to his old established speech pattern, and stutter. He will tend to regress to his old habit of thinking ahead if he happens to have a problem in one or two incidents. This seems to occur regardless of the magnitude of the blocks he may have. When this regression comes, all of the old habits and previous problems return. It may be only a slight "stub of the toe" that turns him around again.

If the person who stutters reverts to his old pattern of thinking ahead, he will stutter again. This happens too often when persons who have known him make a remark, give a look, or offer some other indication that they are aware of his changed speaking behavior. They may make a joke of the manner in which he spoke before and mimic the stuttering. An unthinking person may blurt out the question, "Hey, what happened to your stuttering?" Someone may slap him on the back and say, "Man, you don't stutter anymore." Any of these or similar situations may contain enough suggestion to cause the individual to begin

114

thinking about his speech; this concern can bring back the old habits.

Because of this ever prevailing tendency, the person who has received therapy and is speaking with greater fluency must be cautioned about this possibility. He must be aware that occasionally everyone has a problem with his speech. The former stutterer should not and must not think that his fluent speech is at an end and that he is back to stuttering because of a mishap. He should ignore a difficult encounter and continue to maintain the normal thought-to-speech behavior he has learned. He must stay relaxed and preserve the normal speech breathing patterns. In this way he can continue to conserve the improved, fluent speech he has developed.

The individual who has been through training and has progressed through his hierarchy of difficult speaking situations yet may find new events or one or two old type of encounters that present some problems. He should be advised that this will happen. If at all possible, circumstances permitting, he should rehearse the approaching speaking situation and establish a confident attitude so that he can and will maintain his best speech behaviors.

If any of these occasions arise and stuttering does return, the person immediately should initiate contact with his therapist. The therapist should set up a series of therapy sessions and go through the basic fundamental behaviors of speech that were previously covered. By doing this, it is possible to reestablish quickly the more fluent speaking patterns. The longer he continues to stutter, the more difficult it will be to restore his improved speech behaviors.

Also, the person who stutters should maintain close contact or dependency on the therapist because of the tendency to be discouraged by minor problems that will occur. The association should continue until the more normal speech behaviors have been established permanently, over a long period of time. The therapist must be available for encouragement and/or consultation whenever there is a need, real or imagined. The person who has just completed therapy will need to know that he has support for as long as he may feel the need for it.

At first, the return visits to the therapist should be regularly scheduled appointments, every two weeks or so. The time interval between visits should be lengthened gradually. This type of programmed visitation should be extended to one time a month, once every two months, and eventually to once every six months, or to whatever interval is comfortable for the subject. This schedule should not mean that the individual cannot call in between scheduled appointments if there is need.

MONITORING

Persons who stutter tend to change their speech monitoring to "before the fact rather than after the fact." They are so busy thinking ahead of what they want to say that they are not perceptive of what they are saying. They must learn to monitor their speech correctly, to listen as they speak. It has been said by some of those who stutter that, when they stopped thinking ahead, they became more aware of what they were saying. By monitoring their speech in this more normal sequence pattern of speaking, and hearing it at approximately the same time, some avoid tendencies to think ahead. This process, however, must not become a distraction, or the focal point of their concentration while they are speaking.

The person who stutters should be less critical of himself in the self-monitoring of his speech if he learns to maintain a more normal expectancy of what and how he is speaking. The individual who stutters is not necessarily a perfectionist. He is aware of the variations in his speaking patterns. These variations also tend to be before the fact and not after or during it. He should know that many errors of different varieties can occur while he is speaking. Everyone will mispronounce a word occasionally. People often misarticulate sounds. An individual will even say the wrong thing or be the victim of a "Freudian slip." To make an error in speaking is not an unforgivable sin; it is just being human. The subject should develop a less critical attitude toward his own speech and speaking behavior and join the ranks of the rest of society. Even the best trained and most polished speakers make mistakes.

DELAYED AUDITORY FEEDBACK

For many years there has been considerable interest in delayed auditory feedback and its possible relationship to stuttering. Cherry et al. (1956) suggested that stuttering may be related to an instability of the auditory feedback loop.

To improve understanding of this phenomenon, laboratory experiments have been conducted in which a delay is introduced between what a person is saying and his hearing of it. The individual speaks into a microphone. Earphones are placed over his ears. The volume of the headset is set at a loudness level sufficient to cancel out the speaker's ability to hear and monitor what he is saying. The speaker then hears what has been recorded on a tape and is being played back for him to hear a fraction of a second later than he would normally have heard it. This artificial delay creates much confusion in that, while listening to what he has said over the headset, he must try to continue to speak. Under these circumstances, most persons resort to nonfluent speech, speech that is very characteristic of what occurs in stuttering with numerous clonic and tonic blocks.

This behavior and circumstances is applicable to this author's theory, but on a somewhat different plane. Under delayed auditory feedback, the person hears what he has thought and spoken, while currently thinking of what he is trying to say. The delay in hearing his past thoughts expressed is in conflict with the current thoughts that he is trying to utter. This creates a confusing state of affairs concerning his thought-to-speech behavior.

When a person is thinking ahead of what he wants to say and attempts to continue to express the thoughts he had before, a confusing set of circumstances arises. His speaking and thinking are not concurrent. When thinking ahead occurs, the speaker's attention is on what he is planning to say while he is saying what was thought of a fraction of a second before. This process creates a delay in the expression of current thoughts and causes the same types of nonfluencies as those produced by delayed auditory feedback. The major difference is that those problems created by the delayed feedback are false, or pseudo-stuttering, while the problems that arise as the result of thinking ahead are very real indeed.

The pattern of thinking ahead while speaking appears to create confusion in the neocerebellum. It has received the cortical message to program particular muscle patterns for what is to be said, but the cortex interferes by continuing to relay messages concerning what is to be said. Thus, "thinking ahead," or current thinking, interferes with the expression of past thoughts that the person is trying to speak. Thinking ahead is current thinking; it is what is being thought of now.

In summary, delayed auditory feedback, past thought feedback, interferes with current thought-to-speech behavior and results in pseudo-stuttering. Thinking ahead, current thought, interferes with past thought-to-speech behavior and results in true stuttering behavior.

CHILDHOOD NONFLUENCY

As noted in earlier chapters, stuttering is a childhood phenomenon that has its onset between the ages of two and four years. A possible etiology was presented in Chapter 5. The point of concern now turns to the child who begins to have nonfluencies at this age level. What can and should be done for him or her?

Unfortunately, a child born in the United States, and other countries with similar socioeconomic societies and levels of competition, is going to be subjected to a variety of pressures. These are not of his own making, but are those of his parents, peers, relatives, friends, and neighbors. The hypercritical comparisons and categorizations of what children are doing and should be doing are beyond belief. The differences among children, and what they are doing at various age levels, institute considerable consternation among adults; these differences break up friendships and cause rifts in families.

Under conditions such as these, the child who escapes criticism for nonfluencies is indeed fortunate. Parents and grandparents suffer a deep sense of frustration when the two to four year old member of the family begins talking with nonfluent speech. They immediately decide that something must be done before the problem becomes worse. But what can they do? They seek advice from the family physician, the minister, a friend, or someone else. The most common suggestions are: "Tell him to slow down." "Tell him not to do that," "Make him stop and start over," etc. In addition, the problem is discussed in front of the child.

Throughout the course of normal development, no real concern is generated if the child falls while walking as long as he does not hurt himself. He may knock over his cup of milk, drop food in his lap or on the floor, or swallow his gum to no one's real concern. He makes all kinds of mistakes and blunders his way through a day, but is learning and improving all of the time, and no one becomes distraught. Now, let him have a few nonfluencies, repeat *I* or *me* a few times, and his world comes apart.

This is the result of false information being circulated by all kinds of people through word of mouth, books, newspapers, magazine articles, and all of the various media. Stuttering has become a real stigma in all levels of the child's world and in the socioeconomic society in which he will have to function. He may be barred from certain occupations, the military academies, and some facets of the armed forces. These are but a few of the consequences of the misunderstanding of the problem. The child, and later the adult, will be made to feel the results of this stereotyped thinking and misinformation in the rebuffs he will receive for his nonfluency.

The largest percentage of children who go through this period fortunately do not respond to the looks of concern, the demands to slow down, the chastisements and the mishandling they receive. They do not make the shift in "thinking-to-speech" so readily as do some of their peers, and thus they develop as normal speakers in regard to their fluency of output.

The ideal course of action to take when a child begins to use nonfluent speech is *nothing*. It should be handled as all of the other problems he is having; it is just part of growing and developing. If the parents feel that they must do something, let it be as little as possible. Nothing can be done about the nonfluencies that have just occurred. If the child has more to say, the parent should change the scene and set the pace by remaining calm and collected. The child's attention should be diverted momentarily by suggesting a drink, "come sit down and tell me about it," picking up the child, and continuing the conversation by inserting a slowly stated question, etc. There are many possibilities, depending upon the circumstances. Getting angry and yelling at the child, or showing overconcern, will not help the child at all. The words "stutter," "stuttering," and "stammering" should never be used in the child's presence.

It would be nice if the problem could be handled this easily. Too often, peers or a not too well meaning friend will alert the child to the fact that he has a problem. How seriously he takes the criticism or labeling may determine the extent to which he becomes overly conscious of his thinking and speaking. If the question arises and he asks, "Mom, do I stutter?", the answer must be, "No! I don't know what you are talking about." Then, if absolutely necessary, the parent may have to offer the child an explanation: "You know when you are running, you trip and fall down, or sometimes you drink your milk too fast and spill it all over your chin. Well, those things just happen, but you are getting better." "In talking you 'stub your toe' on a word, but it's all right and you go on talking. You're talking better everyday. As you grow to be a bigger boy, you will do everything better, okay?" The subject then should be changed. All this explanation should be made with a reassuring smile. The child should be held on the parent's lap while this is being discussed.

It is not recommended that this litttle talk be memorized. Every parent knows his or her own child and should know how to paraphrase the above to meet the child's need to understand. It must be done calmly, without a fuss, or an overabundance of concern. Parents should be matter-of-fact about the whole thing, but let the child know that he should not worry about it; stuttering is just one of many phenomena that are happening at this stage of development.

What should be the course of action to be taken if the child continues to have nonfluencies? If the child is having normal nonfluencies, the parent should not seek professional help but rather follow the procedure outlined above. If secondary symptoms appear and the problem appears to be getting worse, and if the child is about five years old, then high quality professional help should be obtained.

After reading this book, the parent is now aware of the problem of stuttering and all of its ramifications. He should use this information when seeking help for his child. What does the therapist know? How does he feel about the problem of stuttering? What therapy program does he follow, if any? What can be expected for the child as the result of the therapy he has to offer? How long will the treatment take? How much will the parent be involved in the program? The parent should not tell what he wants but rather let the therapist tell what he has to offer. He can always say yes to the demands of the parent and not know what the parent is talking about. Is the person a qualified, certified speech pathologist, etc.? What are his credentials?

Do all speech therapists, pathologists, etc., know how to work with and help the child with a stuttering problem? Unfortunately, the answer to this question must be a qualified no!

The trend in the training of speech therapists throughout the country is for public school positions. The reasons given are, "That's where the jobs are and that's where the money is." The therapist must work with a prescribed number of children a week, in some states, perhaps 150. These children are taught primarily in groups of two or three, sometimes more. The sessions are about twenty minutes in length, and are scheduled once or twice a week. These are certainly not the best conditions for working with children who have stuttering problems.

The therapy provided in the public schools and in many clinics throughout the country is directed toward the adaptation effect; some say, behavior modification. Most therapies are centered around play therapy. It is their hope that during play the child will adapt to the situation and begin to speak fluently. He then should carry the fluent speech over into other speaking situations.

In most programs it is suggested that the child speak fluently.

He receives a good mark if he speaks fluently and a bad mark, or no mark at all, if he stutters. The therapist keeps score through period after period of therapy. The child is supposed to learn to speak fluently by way of adaptation and positive reinforcement or reward for good responses, and negative reinforcement for bad responses. In the majority of cases this does not work, and the child continues to stutter, to everyone's consternation. Often, no attempts are made to correct the symptoms or charactertistics of the problem.

It is with regret that this author deemed it necessary to write the preceding paragraphs. If, however, the child who stutters is to receive the help he so drastically needs and the parents are to be directed to quality programs and therapy, the truth must be offered. The problem concerning therapy for adults has reached the point where the Speech Foundation of America (1978) is advising self-therapy in *Self-Therapy for the Stutterer: One Approach*. The therapy recommended is not acceptable to this author's standards.

To the parents: Seek a quality program for your child. If none is available, talk to the most qualified, certified speech therapist in or close to your community. If the answers you receive are not satisfactory according to the standards set forth in this book, recommend that the therapist study this book thoroughly and then decide what he or she can do. Whatever you do, whatever you find, make sure that it meets the needs of your child and his problem. This is a neurophysiological problem and needs to be treated accordingly.

The therapeutic or treatment program suggested for the development of more normal speaking behaviors was given in detail in Chapter 6. In order to visualize the entire program, as it may be used by speech therapists and others qualified to do so, an outline is presented for consideration. It is recommended that each step be considered carefully to achieve the short- and long-term goals that can readily be recognized. The ultimate aim of this program is normal, fluent speech for children and adolescents. Adults will realize varying levels of improvement. This improvement most often will be determined by the desire to speak better and by the strength of the deviant behaviors that have developed. All persons should make some improvement and note a marked reduction in their stuttering.

OUTLINE OF POSSIBLE THERAPY SESSIONS FOR STUTTERING

I. Relaxation
A. Shortened form, assisted
B. Complete relaxation, unassisted

II. Breathing
A. Quiet patterns
   1. Block breathing
   2. Quiet 3:3 patterns
B. Speech breathing
   1. Prolonged *ah*
   2. Series counting
      a. 1 to 4
      b. 1 to 5
      c. 1 to 6
      d. 1 to 7
      e. 1 to 8
   3. Nursery rhymes
   4. Rote questions and answers

III. Basic Principles of Normal Speech
A. Explaining reasons for previously used techniques
   1. Relaxation
   2. Normal breathing patterns
      a. Quiet
      b. Speech
B. Normal thought-to-speech patterns
   1. Don't think ahead
   2. Don't think ahead, just talk, as in using rote material

IV. Rate Control of Speech
A. Speaking to gross motor patterns timed to cardiac rhythms
   1. Tap on the heavy accents in words and sentences

   2. Walk on the heavy accents in words and sentences
B. Duplicating these rhythms without gross motor patterns
C. Material to be used in the foregoing
   1. Nursery rhymes
   2. Prepared sentences
      a. Subject receives articulatory familiarization
      b. Subject prepares sentences for given speech phoneme

V. Working out Hierarchy of the Subject

A. Working through all levels of propositionality: Least pressure to most pressure
B. Preparing for participation through different levels: Rehearsing if necessary

VI. Propositional Speech (Conversational Interaction)

A. Engaging in normal conversation: Subject must maintain all he has learned to this stage
B. Becoming more involved in group discussions

   This is a general outline that may be used to establish a therapy program to meet the needs of the subject. The most important steps are roman numerals I, II, III. These steps form the basis for correcting symptoms and deviant speaking behaviors. They must be basic in any therapeutic program. No attempt should be made to hurry from one step to the next. Each section must be given full consideration, until the therapist feels certain that the person is ready to advance to the next one. The process is designed to build good speaking habits. The total speaking behavior will be only as strong as each basic behavior is strong; weak segments will bring about a collapse of the total speech pattern in time. Modifications in the outline may be needed to meet the variability of the individuals assisted in therapy; their needs must be met.
   One of the most difficult tasks that must be anticipated in working with the adult who stutters is to convince him to work on the various aspects of the program on a consistent basis. Many persons will expect the program to take care of their problems without too much effort on their part. There will be a tendency

for them to want to discontinue therapy before they should do so. They begin to speak more fluently, and for some people this is good enough. The habit of thinking ahead while talking is not an easy one to break; it takes time and a considerable amount of concerted effort to establish the new thought process. The subject needs to be made to realize that the time and effort spent on his program will be very beneficial to him.

SPEECH PROBLEMS RESULTING FORM CEREBELLAR DAMAGE

In Chapter 6 it was noted that the author was convinced that the etiology of stuttering could be correlated with the development of the cerebellum between the ages of two and four years. It was stated that there probably were no lesions or damage to the cerebellum; it was normal. What type or types of speech problems do occur when there is some insult to the cerebellum or the cerebellar tracts?

Dow and Moruzzi (1958) presented some quotes from authors whose manuscripts are not available to this author. The descriptions are of speech problems noted in individuals with damage to the cerebellum or cerebellar tracts. They quoted Holmes (1917) as follows:

> Speech is abnormal in most cases in which the lesions are recent and severe; it is usually slow, drawling and monotonous, but at the same time tends to be staccato and scanning. This gives it an almost typical "singsong" character and makes it indistinct and often difficult to understand. In a few patients speech was in fact unintelligible for a time. In many cases the utterance is remarkably irregular and jerky, and many syllables, especially, as Marie has pointed out, of those that end a sentence, tend to be explosive.
>
> Phonation is as a rule more affected than articulation, though both vowels and consonants are slurred and uttered unequally and irregularly. All classes of consonants, too, are affected but articulation sometimes has a special nasal character and the labials particularly tend to be explosive.
>
> Another striking feature is the apparent effort necessary to utter a series of syllables or a sentence; the attempt is associated with excessive facial grimacing and speech has consequently a laboured character that often recalls pseudobulbar paresis.

Also, they reported that Hillar (1929) "studied the disturb-ance in Friedreich's ataxia and emphasized the influence of poor coordination of respiration and has demonstrated this graphi-cally."

Dow and Moruzzi quoted from Zentay (1937):

> Zentay (1937) has classified the disturbances in speech seen in cere-bellar disorders as follows: (a) ataxic speech, in which articulation, respiration, and phonation may each be interfered with in varying degrees; (b) adiadochokinesis of speech, which he feels expressed it-self in the slowness characteristic of the cerebellar speech disturbances; (c) explosive-hesitant speech, which he feels is due to a disturbance in the "inhibitory or braking" function of the cerebellum; and (d) scan-ning speech, in which there is a stretching of syllables, which are also sharply cut off from one another.

Damage to the cerebellum or cerebellar tracts can result in several types of atxia, one of the five major classifications of cerebral palsy. Ataxia does not relate to stuttering as one of the characteristics of the problem.

Dow and Moruzzi (1958) also reported on the effects of cer-tain exogenous toxins that may affect the Purkinje cells and, therefore, cerebellar function. Among those listed were alcohol and carbon tetrachloride. They stated that the cerebellar cor-tex is one of the most susceptible parts of the nervous system to oxygen deficiency. Vitamin deficiency and nutritional deficits can produce cerebellar symptoms.

None of the above factors appears to cause or be involved in stuttering insofar as it is known by this author to the date of pre-paring this manuscript.

FUTURE STUDY

Neurological and neurophysiological investigation of the cen-tral nervous system, in this instance the cortex and the cerebel-lum, has taken several directions. Ablation experiments have been performed on laboratory animals. Stimulation and electro-physiological experiments have been done on laboratory animals and on some humans in the course of required surgery. The in-formation obtained from these experiments is voluminous.

The results of insults or damage to various parts of the nervous system have been explored extensively. Neurological damage has resulted from all types of traumas of an exogenous nature. Brain or neurological lesions from endogenous insults have resulted from internal diseases of various types, disorders of the cerebrospinal system, cerebrovascular accidents of many varieties, and chromosomal aberrations.

Much of the information known about the function of the central nervous system has been garnered and evaluated as a result of damage to the system. From this information, assumptions have been drawn in regard to how certain areas of the system operate. Exploration and experimentation on human beings is forbidden by law. True laboratory experimentation has to be performed on laboratory animals. The results of animal experiments have been noted and related to humans, often by conjecture. Studies directed toward exploring and understanding the central nervous system of human beings have been going on for years and will need to continue for many years to come. It is not known whether a complete understanding of this complex system will ever be realized. As noted in Chapter 5, there are areas of the cerebellum that have not been explored extensively enough to permit comprehension of this system's complete function; maybe someday this will be achieved.

Future studies in speech science should be directed toward a more complete understanding of the neuromuscular behaviors involved in the problems noted in almost every type of speech disorder. Speech is a neurophysiological and neuromuscular activity. It cannot be anything else. People do talk with their hands and fingers, but normal human communication is by way of oral speech. Speech and language problems can only be dealt with properly and adequately from this point of reference. Research and therapy likewise should follow this progression. The concept that speech is simply a response from the "little black box" (the brain) in response to an environmental stimulus is totally without understanding of how the human being functions. This, however, is the philosophy that forms the basis for many approaches to speech disorders and the development of therapeutic programs. Speech is a true neurophysiological function in all of its ramifications, and no rehabilitative systems can be developed adequately without taking this fact into consideration.

Speech and language form the basis for all human learning. Reading and writing are graphic forms of speech and language. Thinking is done in words and sentences. Visual images are deciphered by the same processes. All sensory stimuli, which reach the conscious level, are decoded by way of speech and language, commonly referred to as thinking. Only in very early infancy and in some conditions where other forms of communication are necessary are stimuli decoded differently, and then, no one is positive that this is not done in some form of speech.

Research on all of the foregoing problems should continue. As an example, the neurophysiology of reading and writing needs exploration. How does it occur? What happens in the nervous system that makes these behaviors possible? Children in public school either read or do not read. Most often the remedies suggested are glasses or ocular muscle training. In many instances these two procedures do not correct the problem. Remedial reading is given to the child, and still he does not read. No one asks or tries to find out why the child is still not reading. He is then said to have a learning disability and more remedial reading is given, similar to that of the previous attempts. Neither medical science nor educational psychology can arrive at the cause of the problem. This is why more research is needed in the field of human learning from a neurophysiological reference. The question arises, How many people in the educational field engaged in teaching the children of this country understand how learning takes place? The standard answer given for a child's not learning is, "He isn't trying hard enough. And this response has not changed in years and years. Those involved in providing services and therapy are too often unaware of what is happening to the human organism as a result of their teaching or programs.

Research is strongly needed to investigate the neurophysiological aspects of human learning. The question is, Will it ever happen? The answer is, Probably not. Neurological scientists are too busy taking care of critical problems and do not have the time. This area on neurophysiological aspects should be thoroughly explored and the results used to upgrade therapies of all types, including education and learning at all levels.

The author has expounded personally through the last few paragraphs. These writings are an outgrowth of the thinking for this book. Human behavior, learning, and personal evaluations of the therapy and treatment given to people, particularly children, have been considered. The recommendations made are the results of observations on therapy and educational processes as provided today; many are lacking in merit and not worth the money expended. Perhaps some of the readers of this book will take note and initiate activities that will prove beneficial to all concerned.

SUMMARY AND CONCLUSIONS

The purpose for writing this manuscript was to relate a new look at stuttering from a neurophysiological viewpoint. Many researchers have suggested a possible relationship, but have not explored it beyond a few superficial possibilities. Most investigators have chosen to fall back on possible psychological or psychiatric etiological assumptions. Some individuals who were very much interested in the neurological and scientific basis of communication and learning are now deceased. In most instances, no one is continuing the work they initiated.

Various therapies have been discussed briefly. Most of the currently used approaches have a psychological orientation and are primarily established on the same basic concepts. A small number of individuals have offered cures for stuttering by working on one or two of the symptoms of the problem. Self-help therapy for those who stutter is receiving encouragement.

Stuttering is a syndrome that is comprised of a complex of symptoms. Some of the symptoms and characteristics of this difficulty are an outgrowth of what a person does to avoid stuttering. Some of the symptoms are the end results of a neurophysiological aberration that appears to be the cause of the continuation of stuttering after the speech should have corrected itself by way of maturation and development of the central nervous system.

Normal childhood nonfluencies appear to result from a developing nervous system in which the cerebellum is not capable of handling the cerebral assignments for prescribed motor behaviors for speech.

Most children tend to become fluent speakers as the cerebellum and central nervous system grow, become myelinated, and mature. The continuation of stuttering may result from a change in thought-to-speech behavior that occurs primarily during the normal nonfluency developmental period. The self-monitoring of speech tends to change from "after the fact to before the fact." Thinking ahead appears to disrupt the integration of the neurophysiological processes for speaking. According to this author, stuttering is a neurophysiological problem that apparently can be corrected.

A therapy or treatment program has been offered. The basic design stresses the correction or remediation of the symptoms and characteristics of stuttering. Therapies of primary concern are relaxation, quiet breathing, speech breathing, and the development of more normal thought-to-speech behaviors. The long-range goal of the therapeutic process is an alteration of the thought-to-speech behavior that is the underlying provocation for the continuation of stuttering.

Childhood stuttering or nonfluency has been considered with recommendations for therapy. Parents have been advised regarding when to seek professional help and how to search for qualified therapists and pathologists.

The higher level language and speech behaviors of reading and writing have been included. These basic mediums of communication are graphic forms of speech and language and should be included as human physiological behaviors.

The emotional aspects of stuttering have been given consideration and compared to similar problems found in other persons with different types of handicaps.

Also, a maintenance program has been suggested for recently acquired or newly learned behaviors. People tend to be remiss in maintaining newly developed motor behaviors and need constant support and encouragement to continue using them.

Finally, childhood normal nonfluencies have been discussed. An acceptable approach in handling this problem has been suggested.

The foregoing paragraphs have been presented as a brief summary of the contents of this manuscript. The hypothesis extended and the therapies recommended have been based on years of clinical experience and a background in neurology, neurophysiology, psychology, speech pathology, audiology, educational psychology, and other related courses. The author has examined and provided therapy for every conceivable type of speech, language, and educational problem, and related disorders. He has had contact with thousands of handicapped persons of all ages and nationalities. He was Chairman of the Neurological Diagnostic Unit of the Institute of Logopedics in Wichita, Kansas, from its inception until it was disbanded as such in 1972. (The staff neurologist, an M.D., took another position and thus terminated the integrity of the unit.) This author also served as the Principal Speech Pathologist for the Unit.

With this background, and other experiences not related here, the author strongly supports what has been written in this manuscript. The search for this hypothesis has been carried on for over a quarter century. A multitude of avenues have been explored. The final connecting pieces of the problem did not become apparent until a few years ago. The pieces of the stuttering puzzle now seem to fit so as to form a logical picture that encompasses all of the ramifications of the problem.

This presentation may not be the complete picture of the problem of stuttering, but it is felt that it may be a logical step toward a solution to the problem. The etiology of stuttering appears to be neurophysiological. The continuation of stuttering seems to be caused by an alteration in neurophysiological behavior that continues to interfere with the normal processes of thinking and speaking.

There will be many persons who will take issue with what has been written here; that is their privilege. It is hoped that the criticisms will be of a constructive nature and will not be blatant rejections of all that has been offered. All that the author asks is that the reader approach the material presented with an open mind, and give full consideration to the facts and logic that support the hypothesis. It is requested that the therapies be tried and evaluated honestly before they are condemned.

As stated earlier, it is not proposed that this hypothesis, which relates the cause of stuttering to the lack of cerebellar development and its interaction to a change in thought-to-speech behavior, and the therapeutic program be considered the final words concerning the problem of stuttering. It is hoped that this work has awakened new interests and thinking concerning stuttering behavior. May the theory presented revitalize research and experimentation by all health-related fields interested in this speech disorder. It will have been more than worth the time and effort expended in its preparation if this writing initiates further investigation into the neurophysiology of stuttering and other human behaviors and results in improved rehabilitation for all of those involved.

GLOSSARY

Anxiety: A feeling of apprehension, uncertainty, and fear.

Archicerebellum: The earliest developed portion of the cerebellum.

Athetoid, athetosis: A form of cerebral palsy characterized by the presence of constant, involuntary, choreiform like motions.

Axon: The essential conduction part of a nerve fiber.

Cardiac rhythms: Rhythms of the heart; the pulse beat is taken as the basic cardiac rhythm.

Cerebellum: That division of the brain behind the cerebrum and above the pons and fourth ventricle. It consists of a median lobe and two lateral lobes, connected with the other portions of the brain by three pairs of peduncles: the superior with the cerebrum, the middle with the pons, and the inferior with the medula. It is concerned with the coordination of movements.

Cerebral: Pertaining to the cerebrum: the main portion of the brain occupying the upper part of the cranium, the two cerebral hemispheres, united by the corpus callosum, forming the largest part of the central nervous system in man.

Cerebral palsy: Any one of a group of conditions affecting control of the motor system, due to lesions in various parts of the brain and occurring as a result of birth injury or prenatal cerebral defect.

Compulsion neurotic: A mental disorder characterized by an irresistible impulse to perform a morbid act or an act considered morbid by the subject.

Cortex, cerebral: The cortex of the brain, composed mainly of gray or cineritious substance; cortex, the outer layer of an organ as distinguished from its inner substance.

Ego: In psychoanalytic psychology, the ego is that part of the psychic apparatus that is the mediator between the person and reality; its prime function is the perception of reality and adaptation to it.

Endocrine: Secreting internally; applicable to organs whose function is to secrete into the blood or lymph a substance that has a specific effect on another gland or part.

Exhalation: The expelling of air from the lungs by breathing.

Expiration: The act of breathing out or expelling air from the lungs or chest.

Hypothalamus: The portion of the diencephalon that forms the floor and part of the lateral wall of the third ventricle. The nuclei of this region exert control over visceral functions involving the autonomic nervous system. Functions include regulation of sexual activity, water, fat and carbohydrate metabolism, and heat regulation.

Inhalation: The drawing of air or other vapor into the lungs.

Inspiration: The act of drawing air into the lungs.

Intrapsychic: Situated, originating, or taking place within the psyche.

Kinesiology: The sum of what is known about human motion.

Limbic system: This term is replacing rhinencephalon, which should be reserved for structures concerned with the sense of smell, although smell has a strong emotional impact, readily evokes disgust or relish, and is powerful in awakening emotional associations. Hippocampus of the limbic system has been reported as contributing to emotional responses that cannot be conditioned without it; it discharges chiefly to the hypothalamus and epithalamus.

Muscles, skeletal: Striated muscles that are attached to the bones: striated; striped: any muscles whose fibers are divided by transverse striations; such muscles are voluntary.

Myelinate, myelinization: The act of taking on myelin, the fat-like substance forming a sheath around certain nerve fibers; noted to be essential for the propagation of nervous impulses.

Neocerebellum: The later developed part of the cerebellum, comprising the lateral lobes and dentate nucleus.

Neurology: That branch of medical science that deals with the nervous system, both normal and in disease.

Neuromuscular: Pertaining to nerves and muscles.

Neurophysiology: The physiology of the nervous system; physiology: the science which treats of the functions of the living organism and its parts.

Neurotic behavior: Affected by neurosis: seen in a person in whom emotions predominate over reason. Symptoms of neurosis include sensory, motor, or visceral disturbances and mental disturbances such as anxieties, specific fears and avoidances, memory disturbances, trance states, somnambulisms, troublesome thoughts, and the like.

Organic: Pertaining to an organ or the organs: the part of the body having a special function.

Paleocerebellum: The earlier formed part of the cerebellum, comprising the vermis and the flocculus and a part of the cerebellar hemispheres.

Parasympathetic nervous system: The cranoisacral division of the autonomic nervous system, which is made up of the occular division, the bulbar division, and the sacral division.

Psychotic: Pertaining to, characterized by, or caused by psychosis; psychosis is the deeper, more far-reaching and prolonged behavior disorder, such as dementia praecox and manic-depressive.

Respiration: The act or function of breathing.

Sympathetic nervous system: One of the two subdivisions of the autonomic nervous system arising from the lateral gray column in the thoracic and upper lumbar segments of the spinal cord. In general, if the sympathetic division excites or fortifies an activity, the parasympathetic will inhibit it, and vice versa. It prepares the organism for fight or flight. It speeds up the heart to distribute oxygen and metabolites for emergency, etc.

Synergy: In neurology, the faculty by which movements are properly grouped for the performance of acts requiring special adjustments.

REFERENCES

Andrews, Gavin and Harris, Mary: *The Syndrome of Stuttering.* London, Spastics International Medical, 1964.

Barbara, Dominick A.: *The Psychotherapy of Stuttering.* Springfield, Thomas, 1962.

Berry, Mildred F. and Eisenson, Jon: *Speech Disorders. Principles and Practices of Therapy.* New York, (Appleton), Prentice-Hall, 1956.

Bloodstein, Oliver: Conditions under which stuttering is reduced or absent: A review of the literature. *JSHD, 14:*295, 1949.

———: Hypothetical conditions under which stuttering is reduced or absent. *JSHD, 15:*142–153, 1950.

———: Stuttering as an anticipatory struggle reaction. In Eisenson, Jon (Ed.): *Stuttering: A Symposium.* New York, Harper and Row, 1958.

———: The development of stuttering, I. Changes in nine basic features. *JSHD, 25:*219, 1960a.

———: The development of stuttering, II. Developmental phases. *JSHD, 25:*366, 1960b.

———: The development of stuttering, III. Theoretical and clinical implications. *JSHD, 26:*67, 1961.

Bryngelson, Bryng: A study of laterality of stutterers and normal speakers. *Speech, 4(3):*231–234, 1939.

———: Stuttering and personality development. *The Nervous Child, 2,* 1943.

Cherry, E. Colin and Mc-A. Sayers, Bruce: Human cross correlator, a technique for measuring certain parameters of speech perception. *J Acoust Soc Am, 28(5):*889–895, 1956.

Dorland, W.A. Newman, et al.: *Dorland's Illustrated Medical Dictionary,* 23rd ed. Philadelphia, Saunders, 1957.

Dow, Robert Stone and Moruzzi, Giuseppe: *The Physiology and Pathology of the Cerebellum.* Minneapolis, University Press, 1958.

Dunlap, Knight: The technique of negative practice. *Am J Psychol, 55:* 270–273, 1932.

Eisenson, Jon: A perseverative theory of stuttering. In Eisenson, Jon (Ed.): *Stuttering: A Symposium.* New York, Harper and Row, 1958.

Eisenson, Jon: (*See* Berry and Eisenson, 1956.)

Elliott, H. Chandler: *Textbook of Neuroanatomy,* 2nd ed. Philadelphia, Lippincott, 1969.

Fay, Temple: Speech analysis, a cornerstone in the rehabilitation of language. *Cerebral Palsy Rev*, January-February, 1953.

Fraser, Malcolm: *Self-therapy for the Stutterer: One Approach.* Memphis, Speech Foundation of America, 1978.

Glauber, I. Peter: The psychoanalysis of stuttering. In Eisenson, Jon (Ed.): *Stuttering: A Symposium.* New York, Harper and Row, 1958.

Goldiamond, Israel: Experiment wipes out stuttering. *Wichita* [Kansas] *Eagle,* Associated Press, Chicago, 1974.

Grinker, Roy R. and Bucy, Paul C.: *Neurology,* 4th ed. Springfield, Thomas, 1949.

Hinsie, Leland E. and Campbell, Robert J.: *Psychiatric Dictionary,* 4th ed. New York, Oxford University Press, 1971.

Howell, William H.: *A Textbook of Physiology.* John F. Fulton (Ed.): Philadelphia, Saunders, 1949.

Jacobson, Edmund: *Progressive Relaxation: A Physiological and Clinical Investigation of Muscular States and Their Significance in Psychology and Medical Practice,* 2nd ed. Chicago, University of Chicago Press,

Johnson, Wendell and Knott, John R.: Studies in psychology of stuttering: 1 the distribution of moments of stuttering in successive readings of the same material. *JSHD,* 2:17–19, 1937.

Johnson, Wendell: Role of evaluation in stuttering behavior. *JSHD, 3:* 85–94, 1939.

———: Study of the onset and development of stuttering. *JSHD, 7(3):*251–258, 1942.

Kanner, Leo: *Child Psychiatry,* 3rd ed. Springfield, Thomas, 1957.

Karlin, Isaac W.: Stuttering, the problem today. *JAMA, 143(8):*732–736, 1950.

Palmer, Martin F.: The cardiac cycle as a physiological determinant in energy distributions in speech. *Speech Monographs,* December, 1937.

———: Synchronization of the events of the cardiac with the onsets of respiratory movements. *JSHD, 4:4,* 375–380, 1942.

———: Class notes. Lectures on stuttering, Wichita University, 1951.

Palmer, Martin F. and Gillett, Anna Mae: Sex differences in cardiac rhythms of stutterers. *JSHD, 4:*133–140, 1938.

———: Respiratory arrhythmia in stuttering. *JSHD, 4(2):*133–140, 1939.

Ruch, T.C.: Basal ganglia and cerebellum. In Ruch, T.C. et al. (Eds.): *Neurophysiology,* 2nd ed. Philadelphia, Saunders, 1965.

Schwartz, Martin F.: *Stuttering Solved.* New York, McGraw-Hill, 1976.

Sheehan, Joseph C.: Theory and treatment of stuttering as an approach avoidance conflict. *J Psychol, 36:*27, 1953.

———: Conflict theroy of stuttering. In Eisenson, Jon (Ed.): *Stuttering: A Symposium.* New York, Harper and Row, 1958.

Snider, R.S. and Stowell, A.: Receiving areas of tactile, auditory and visual systems in the cerebellum. *J Neurophysiol, 7:*331, 1944.

Stein, Leopold: Stammering as a psychosomatic disorder. *Folia Phoniatr,* 5:12–46, 1953.

Travis, Lee E.: My present thinking on stuttering. *Western Speech, 10:* 3–5, 1946.

Travis, Lee E. and Knott, John R.: Bilaterally recorded brain potentials from normal speakers and stutterers. *JSHD, 2(2):*239–241, 1937.

Travis, Lee E. and Lindsley, Donald: An action current study of handedness in relation to stuttering. *J Exp Psychol, 16(2):*258–270, 1933.

Van Dantzig, Marijn: Syllable tapping: New method for the help of stammering. *JSHD, 5(2):*127–132, 1940.

Van Riper, Charles: *Speech Correction: Principles and Methods,* 3rd ed. New York, Prentice-Hall, 1954.

——: Experiments in stuttering therapy. In Eisenson, Jon (Ed.): *Stuttering: A Symposium.* New York, Harper and Row, 1958.

West, Robert W.: An agnostic's speculations about stuttering. In Eisenson, Jon (Ed.): *Stuttering: A Symposium.* New York, Harper and Row, 1958.

West, Robert W. and Ansberry, Merle: *The Rehabilitation of Speech,* 4th ed. New York, Harper and Row, 1968.

Wichita [Kansas] *Eagle and Beacon.* September 27, 1977.

Wischner, George J.: Stuttering behavior and learning: A preliminary theoretical formulation. *J Speech Hear Disord, 15:*324–335, 1950.

INDEX

A

A new look at the old problem, 59-75
Adults, therapy problems with (*see* Therapy, adult problems)
Alingering, stuttering, as (*see* Stuttering, alingering behavior in)
Andrews, Gavin, 7-8
Ansberry, Merle, 76
Anticipation, stuttering and (*see* Stuttering, anticipation in)
Anticipatory struggle reaction (*see* Stuttering, an etiology of)
Anxiety
  guilt and (*see* Guilt)
  intrapsychic, 20
  learned reaction system of, stuttering as a (*see* Stuttering, an etiology of)
  motivation of stuttering by, 17
  physiological type of, 37
  psychological type of, 37
  somatic type of, 37
Approach-avoidance, levels of (*see* Stuttering, approach-avoidance)
Aristotle, 3

B

Bloodstein, Oliver, 15, 16, 17, 47
Boland, John L., 48
Breathing, 87-101
  block, 90, fig. 90
  deviant quiet, therapy for, 90-92
  normal and stuttering patterns of, comparison of, 30-31, 52-53
  normal process of, 73-74
  polygraph and kymograph recordings of, 52
  quiet, normal, 87, fig. 88
  quiet, stuttering persons, 52-53, 73-74, 88-89, fig. 89

speech, fluent speaker's, 92-93, fig. 93
speech, program for normalizing, 96-99
speech, stuttering person's, 52-53, 73-74, 93-95, fig. 93, 95
Bryngelson, Bryng, 29, 41
Bucy, Paul C., 63

C

Cardiac rhythms, stuttering and normal person's (*see* Stuttering, cardiac rhythms in)
Central nervous system and stuttering (*see* Stuttering, central nervous system in)
Cerebellum
  asynergic syndrome of, 63
  cerebral cortex and, connections between, 65-66, 66-69
  cerebral cortex and, speech and functions of, 66-69, 74
  computed motor behaviors from, 66
  correlation center of the, 64
  exogenous toxins on, effects of, 126
  functions of, past considerations of, 64
  functions of, recent considerations of, 64-66
  growth of, motor development and the, 68-69
  neocerebellum of the, functions of the, 64-65
  neocerebellum of the, voluntary motor behavior by, control of, 11
  normal nonfluencies and the, development of, 69
  paleocerebellum of the, 65, 68
  programming by the, speech, 74
  speech and the, development of, 68-69

speech problems and the (*see* Speech, problems of, cerebellar damage and)

stuttering and the, development of, 71

stuttering and the, new look at the onset of (*see* Stuttering, onset of)

synergic control of speech patterns by, 68-69

three developmental-functional divisions of, 68

three regions of, 64-65

voluntary motor responses programmed in, 66

voluntary movement, synergic control of, 63, 64

Cerebral cortex
association areas of, 64-69
investigations of, 126-127

Cerebral hemispheres, control of speech functions by, 28

Cerebral palsy
propositional disorders in (*see* Propositionality, cerebral palsy and)
stuttering and (*see* Stuttering, cerebral palsy and)

Cerebro-cerebellar pathways (*see* Cerebellum, cerebral cortex and)

Cherry, E. Colin, 43, 117

Childhood
nonfluencies in (*see* Nonfluencies, childhood)
stuttering in (*see* Stuttering, childhood stuttering)
stuttering in, therapy for (*see* Therapy, childhood stuttering)

Clonic blocks, repetition as (*see* Stuttering, clonic blocks in)

Clonus, definition of (*see* Stuttering, definition of, clonus in the)

Cluttering (*see* Stuttering versus cluttering)

Computer, human brain as a, 79

Conflict, approach-avoidance (*see* Stuttering, an etiology of)

Cortical speech areas, myelinization of, 27

D

Desensitization (*see* Therapy, stuttering, behavior modification in)

Diabetes, incidence of stuttering in (*see* Stuttering, diabetes in)

Diagnosogenic theory (*see* Stuttering, an etiology of)

Distraction (s)
breathing as a, 98
cautions concerning, 80
rate control of speech as a, 103
use of, oppositions to the, 38
use of, therapeutic, 38

Dollard, J., 22

"Don't think, just talk," 112

Dorland's medical dictionary, 7, 8, 26, 50, 76

Dow, Robert S., 125-126

Dunlap, Knight, 41

E

Easter seal rehabilitation center, 43

Egypt, 3

Eisenson, Jon, 26-27, 41-42

Elliott, H. Chandler, 63, 64, 65, 66, 68

Emotional problems
stuttering caused by, no proof, 31-32
stuttering, other speech handicaps and, 31-32

Emotional stress (*see* Stress)

Emotions, 54
guilt, stuttering and (*see* Guilt)
stuttering persons and, 110-111

Encephalitis, stuttering and (*see* Stuttering, an etiology of)

Endocrine system, stuttering and the (*see* Stuttering, an etiology of)

Epilepsy, stuttering and (*see* Stuttering, an etiology of)

F

Fay, Dr. Temple, 11, 69

Feedback, auditory delayed (*see* Auditory feedback, delayed)

Fluent and nonfluent periods of speech (*see* Stuttering, cycling phenomenon in)

Future study, indications for, 126-129

G

Galen, 3
Glauber, I. Peter, 19-20, 39
Goldiamond, Israel, 43
Gregory, Hugo L., 44
Grinker, Roy R., 63
Guilt
  anxieties and, stuttering, 24
  reactions of stutterers to, 23

H

Habits, human actions as, 79
Harris, Mary, 7
Herodotus, 3
Hippocrates, 3
Howell, William H., 92
Human learning
  basis for (*see* Learning, human)
  investigation of (*see* Learning, human)
Hypertonus, 53

J

Jacobson, Edmund, 80
Johnson, Wendell B., 14-15, 41

K

Kanner, Leo, 21
Karlin, Isaac W., 27-28

L

Laryngeal valving and stuttering, 51-52
Learning
  a philosophy of, 78
  human, basis for, 128
  human, investigation of, 128
Luper, Harold L., 44

M

MacKeith, R., 24
Monitoring, 116
Moses, 3
Mowrer, O.H., 17
Muscle behavior, coordination in articulate speech by (*see* Speech, articulation of)

N

Nervous system, central
  gross lesions in, anatomical dysfunctions and, 32
  mechanics of speech by, 32
  motor activities by, control of, 63
  reprogramming of, 78
  thalamo-cortico-stria pathways of, stuttering and, 32
Neocerebellum, 63 (*see also* Cerebellum)
Neurological complications, stuttering and (*see* Stuttering, an etiology of)
Neurological transmission of thought to speech, 77
Neuromuscular patterns in stuttering (*see* Stuttering, neuromuscular patterns in)
Neurophysiology, cerebellum and cerebral cortex (*see* cerebellum and)
Neurophysiological-physiological variations as the result of stuttering (*see* Stuttering, neurophysiological-physiological)
Neurophysiology, stuttering caused by (*see* Stuttering, an etiology of)
Nonfluency, childhood, 118-123
  basis of, 60-64
  continuation of, a new look at the, 74-75
  handling, recommended procedures for, 119-120
  normal fluency and, 109-110
  normal, parental guidance for coping with, 121-122
Normal fluent speech, development of (*see* Speech)

P

Paleocerebellum, functions of (*see* cerebellum)
Palmer, Dr. Martin F., 11, 29-32, 81, 90
Parents, a message to (*see* Nonfluencies, childhood)
Pavlov, 5
Perseveration
  definition of, 26

organic form of, 26
psychological, a form of, 26
stuttering as a manifestation of, 26
Propositionality
cerebral palsy and, 30
effects of, normal speech and the, 9-10
levels of, extension of the, 108-109
stuttering and levels of, 72
stuttering related to, 30
Psychiatric dictionary, 20, 37
Psychoanalytic theory of stuttering (*see* Stuttering, an etiology of)
Psychological conflict, stuttering as a (*see* Stuttering, an eitology of)
Psychoneurotic conflict, stuttering as a (*see* Stuttering, an etiology of)
Pyknolepsy, stuttering as a form of (*see* Stuttering, an etiology of)

R
Reading
communication and, 104
problems in, 128
Reflex, airway dilation, 28
Relaxation, muscle, 80-87
arm, 83, 85
facial, 83-84, 86
leg, 82, 84
neck, 83, 86
Palmer recommended, 81-84
progressive, 80-81
respiratory, 84, 87
shortened form of, 84-87
shoulder, 82, 85
trunk, 83, 86
Ruch, T.C., 64

S
Schwartz, Martin F., 28-29, 43-44
Secondary symptoms, 22, 36, 54-56, 72-73, 104-105
distractions become, 56
elimination of (*see* Therapy, secondary symptoms)
Self therapy for stuttering, 44-45
Semantics, melody, rhythm and accent in, 102-103
Sheehan, Joseph C., 22-23
Simon, Dr. Clarence, 11

Singing, no stuttering in (*see* Stuttering, singing without)
Snider, R.S., 64
Speech
anticipations during, 9-10
articulation of, 77-78, 101-102
ataxic (*see* Ataxia)
breathing for, (*see* Breathing)
breathing problems in (*see* Breathing)
cerebellar and cortical interactions in, 66-69, 74, 77-78
childhood, development of, 4, 60-63, 66-69
development of, cerebellum and (*see* Cerebellum)
energy in, physiological determinants of, 29-30
fluency and nonfluency in, 109-110
fluent, development of, 4 (*see also,* Speech, development of)
melody, rhythm and accent in, 102-103
monitoring of, 116
muscle behaviors of, development of, 62
neurophysiology of, 67
nonfluent, normal childhood (*see* Nonfluencies, Childhood)
normal
definition of, 76-77
mechanics of, 99
propositionality in, 9
stuttering and, comparison of, 9-10
therapy program for establishing (*see* Therapy, normal speech through)
maintenance of (*see* Therapy, maintenance of)
normalized, relapse of, 114-115
problems of, cerebellar damage and, 125-126
production of, cerebellar programming of, 66-69, 74
programmed as, muscle behavior, 67
rate control of, 102-103
rate of, stuttering person's, 57
stuttering, propositionality and fluency in, 9, 109-110

vital capacity for (*see* Breathing)
voluntary muscle behavior in, 67
Speech defect, stuttering as five characteristics of, 25
Speech doubters, stutterers as, 22
Speech Foundation of America, 43, 122
Speech, thought to, 70-74, 77
  changes in, stuttering person's, 12, 70-71
  duration of time in, normal speakers, 70
Speech science, future studies in, 127-128
Stein, Leopold, 20-21
Stowell, A., 64
Stress
  conditioned reflex of, 29
  definition of, 37
  emotional reaction to, 21
  stuttering and emotional, 28
Stuttering
  alingering behavior in, 25
  ambilateral control of speech in, 29
  anal-sadistic reactions in, 20
  anticipation in, effects of, 9-10, 106-107
  athetosis and, comparison of, 30
  behavior in, thought to speech, 12, 70-72, 74-75, 77, 106-107
  behavior in, learned anxiety reaction, 17
  breathing and (*see* Breathing)
  cardiac rhythms in, comparison of normal, 31
  central nervous system in, changes in, 24
  cerebral palsy and, 24, 30
  clonic blocks in, 8-9, 25, 51
  consequences of, 118-119
  cycling phenomenon in, 74-75 (*see also* Stuttering, childhood)
  diabetes in, incidence of, 31
  emotional problems in (*see* Emotions)
  emotional stress and (*see* Stress)
  emotional vulnerability in, 21
  endocrine system and (*see* Stuttering, an etiology of)
  fluency disruptors in, 32

fluency in, propositionality and, 9
  (*see also*, Propositionality)
  four types of, Schwartz's, 29
  history of, 3
  muscle tension in (*see* Hypertonus)
  neurological-physiological variations and, 23, 32
  neuromuscular patterns in, 8-9
  no correction for, 5, 6, 7
  normal speech and, comparison of, 9
  onset of (*see* Stuttering, onset of)
  perpetuation of, 17, 18, 33, 70-74
  precipitation of, anxiety and guilt in the, 24
  primary and secondary, distinction between, 33
  primary questions concerning, 10
  propositionality and (*see* Propositionality)
  sex differences in, 31
  singing without, 9, 72
  speech breathing patterns in (*see* Breathing)
  stammering and, 7
  symptom complex of, 8, 9, 12, 37, 58
  symptoms of
    reduction of, 47
    reinforcement of, 33
  thalamo-cortico-stria pathways in (*see* Nervous system, central)
  therapy for (*see* Therapy, stuttering)
  thinking ahead and, 12, 71, 72, 73, 74, 106-107
  tics in, 25-26
  tonic blocks in, 8, 25, 51
  tonus in, 8
Stuttering as a speech problem, 9, 25, 50
Stuttering blocks
  tonic and clonic (*see* Stuttering, clonic; tonic)
  unspeakable thoughts and feelings in, 28
Stuttering, an etiology of,
  anticipatory struggle reaction as, 15-16
  anxiety reaction system as, learned, 17

approach-avoidance as, 22-23
atavistic heredity as, 24
auditory feedback as, delayed, 43
author's theory concerning, 11-12
brain injury as, 24
delayed myelinization of cortical
  speech areas, 27
diagnosogenic theory as, 14
ego-id conflict as, 19-20
encephalitis as, 23
endocrine system as, 31
epilepsy as, 24-25
hysteroid dysfluencies as, 24, 25
imitation as, learned, 27
irregular breathing patterns do
  not cause, 53
learned behavior as, theory of, 14
lesions as, no gross neurological, 32
neurological complications as, 27
neurophysiology base, 8, 11-12
neurotic and psychotic conflict as, 7
neurotic behavior as, 21
oral fixation, 20, 25
parents labeling as, 14, 33
pathophysiological subsoil in, 28
psychiatrists suggest, 4
psychogenic base as, 27
psychological conflict as, 19-23
psychologists suggest, 4
psychoneurotic conflict as, 19-23
pyknolepsy as, 25
reflex as, airway dilation, 28-29
speech pathologists and scientists
  suggest, 4-5
unsuccessful gratification of needs
  as, 28
Stuttering, childhood (*see also* Nonfluencies, childhood)
cause of, 60-63
child who becomes, course of action
  for handling (*see* Nonfluencies
  childhood)
children who become, 32-33
continuation of, after 4 to 5 years,
  5, 12, 70-71
fluent and nonfluent cycles in, 36
mistaking normal nonfluency as,
  118-119
parent labeling as a cause of, 14

therapy for (*see* Therapy, childhood
  stuttering)
Stuttering, definitions of
Andrews and Harris, 7-8
author's, 9
clonus and tonus in the, 8
neurophysiological, 8
Stuttering, development of
role of the cerebellum in, 68-71 (*see
  also* Cerebellum)
phases in the, 16
Stuttering, neurophysiology of, 8 (*see
  also* Cerebellum)
a comparison, of differences with
  normals in, 30
Stuttering, onset of (*see also* Stuttering, prevailing theories of)
accepted ages for, 32, 70
nature of the, 4, 5
new look at the, 69-72
peaks of, 31
Stuttering, prevailing theories of, 14-34
Stuttering, remediation of (*see* Therapy, stuttering)
Stuttering, secondary symptoms in
  (*see* Secondary symptoms)
Stuttering, solved, 28-29, 43-44
Stuttering, speech in, monitoring of,
  116
Stuttering, speech rate of (*see* Speech,
  rate of)
Stuttering versus cluttering, 56-58
Summary and conclusions, 129-132

T

Theories, stuttering (*see* Stuttering,
  an etiology of)
Theories, symptoms as basis for, 60
Theory, author's, 10-12, 59-75
Therapy, stuttering
adaptation in, 122
adult problems in, 112, 122, 124-125
airflow techniques in, 44
articulation in, 101-102
auditory delayed feedback in, 43
avoidance tendencies in, reduction
  of, 39
behavior modification in, 45-47
change of handedness in, 45

childhood, guide for finding, 120-
122
childhood, psychological methods in,
19, 39, 40
choral reading in, 45
correction of stuttering through, 43
differences in, adult and childhood,
111-112
distractions in, use of, 38
four objectives of, 41
hierarchies in, 46, 108-109
hypnosis in, use of, 40
maintenance of fluency after, 114-
116
major emphasis today in, 48
melody, rhythm and accent in (*see*
Speech)
negative practice in, 41, 105
normal speech through, 79
outline of sessions in, 123-124
play therapy in, 121
practice materials for, 99-100
procedures for, 12
psychoanalytic, 39
psychotherapy in, 39-40
public school, 121-122
questions concerning, 121
quiet breathing in (*see* Breathing)
rate control in (*see* Speech, rate
control of)
rationale for, 42
reading in, 104
recommendations for, 121-122
relapse of speech after, 114-115
relationship, 40
relaxation in, 44 (*see also* Relaxation)
results of, 112

secondary symptoms in, elimination
of, 104-105
self-help, 43
speech breathing in (*see* Breathing)
syllable tapping in, 47
symptomatic and psychotherapy in,
42
symptoms as, elimination of, 60
symptoms in, reduction of, 47
therapists capabilities to provide,
121
thinking ahead in, elimination of,
106-107
voluntary stuttering in, 41
Thinking aloud, 106-107
Thought patterns, stuttering and normal (*see* Speech, thought to)
Tics, stutterer's, evolution of (*see*
Stuttering, tics in)
Tonic blocks, stoppages as (*see* Stuttering, tonic blocks)
Travis, Lee E., 28, 45
Treatments, stuttering, seven suggested, 6 (*see* Therapy, stuttering)

V
Van Dantzig, Marijn, 47
Van Kirk, 43
Van Riper, Charles, 32-33, 42, 43
Voluntary muscle behavior, speech as
a (*see* Speech, voluntary muscle be-
havior in)

W
West, Robert W., 24-26, 76
Wishner, George J., 17, 18

Z
Zentay, 126